HUGIN MUNIN

GOD'S MENTAL MEDICINE CHEST – THE WORKBOOK

BASED ON THE RUSSIAN CURES (E.G. GRIGORI GRABOVOI)

– Mysteries of the cure

– Psychological standardization

– Powerful healing pictures of the reincarnation of Leonardo da Vinci

– The guide-line of recovery and excellent self-development

Jelezky Publishing, Hamburg 2014

Jelezky Publishing, Hamburg

www.jelezky-publishing.com

First English Edition, June 2014

© 2014 English Language Edition

Edition: 2014-1, 15.06.2014

SVET UG, Hamburg (Publisher)

Published by SVET UG, Hamburg, Germany 2014

For further information on the contents of this book contact:

SVET Centre, Hamburg

www.svet-centre.com

ISBN: 978-3-943110-78-4

According to the responses we have received, the contents of this book have helped many people. We are confident that this will continue to be the case.

Nonetheless, we would like to point out that the techniques of Grigori Grabovoi are mental methods for the guidance of events in one's life. These methods are dependent upon one's personal spiritual development. Because we are dealing with topics relating to one's health, we give this express notice that such influence is not a "therapy" in the conventional sense of the word and is therefore not intended to limit or replace professional medical care.

When in doubt, follow the directions of your doctor or a therapist or pharmacist whom you trust!
(When following conventional methods, you must expect to get conventional results.)

Disclaimer:
The information within this book is intended as reference material only, and not as medical or professional advice.

Information contained herein is intended to give you the tools to make informed decisions about your lifestyle. It should not be used as a substitute for any treatment that has been prescribed or recommended by your qualified doctor. Do not stop taking any medication unless advised by your qualified doctor to do otherwise. The author and publisher are not healthcare professionals, and expressly disclaim any responsibility for any adverse effects occurring as a result of the use of suggestions or information in this book. This book is offered for your own education and enjoyment only. As always, never begin a health program without first consulting a qualified healthcare professional. Your use of this book indicates your agreement to these terms.

Jelelezky Publishing/SVET Centre, Hamburg

„Dear Reader,

Hugin Munin describes in his works my technologies and methods in an extended way. This makes it easier to practice for many people.

Hugin Munin understands exactly the indicated concentrations and thoughts which are outlined in my works. And he transfers his knowledge precisely. He sees the deep interactions of my methods to the wholeness of all external and internal information. And he also sees the interactions to the technology for realization of the control of aims. This gives immediately the integral practice of the development of rescue and eternal life.

Kind regards
Grigori Grabovoi   21-4-2014"

„Dear Reader,

The today living re-incarnation of a gifted painter like Leonardo da Vinci works with information influencing materia. If the painter is in his mental creativity, then God is mirrorring himself.in the pictures with all the qualities God owns. Contemplating on a painting created in such a way, brings us impulses for our eternity and for our development of an eternal life. The paintings in this book have been created by Sergey Jelezky. He is – according to Grigori Grabovoi – the re-incarnation of Leonardo da Vinci. So please take your time to look carefully at these pictures. The painter got the task to create a help for those who need help. He was asked e.g. for a painting helping in case of severe disease. The painter himself asked for spiritual support and got the answer. If you look at the paintings you see the result.

Hugin Munin" 5-5-2014

CHECKLISTS, CLEAR STEP SEQUENCES, AVOIDANCE OF NON-SUCCESS

• What clairvoyants see while healing.

• How you can guarantee with the guide structure to consider all phases of recovery in the right order.

• How you can help yourself and others step by step with every exercise with clear step sequences.

• How you can find the best method for your problem/ your illness.

• How you can find the right alternative methods of a phase.

• How you can use this book as a reference work and find the sought-after method within 40 seconds.

• How you can create yourself an own space/time area and which advantages you will have through this.

• How you can build up with 18 methods a quality such as clairvoyance.

• How you can escape from <u>heavy</u> dark problems/ energies which can block your cure.

• How you can assure the conditions for your cure.

• How you can use the **healing pictures** of the reincarnation of

Leonardo da Vinci.

• How you can raise the **New Consciousness** within yourself.

Whoever carries this book with himself, is already working on his health.
<u>Because:</u> the building-up system of the texts of Grigori Grabovoi is already working alone from the texts within a radius of 5 meters. We should direct our thoughts to Grigori Grabovoi.
Use this book as a standard reference work on the New Age.

INDEX:

PREFACE:

Please let`s don`t fool ourselves. **Who does not want to be successful?** To succeed is nothing obscene. **This applies to all issues**, whether for professional, economic, social, health or mental issues. **The variety of the methods which promise us success are much more doubtful.**

There are enough **esoteric schools and „scientific" methods** with great promises on the market. **Have you ever thought before why there are so many of them and why they often cause so little?** Rudolf Steiner has already taken position to the esoteric schools 100 years ago. He has forecasted exactly what we are now experiencing. The variety exists to confuse us. Whoever puts this variety into the world tries to make a good job of it. It is clear: If the non-rational train can`t be stopped anymore, then so many tracks will be installed at the junction plate until no one knows anymore how it works.

And the science?

If we look exactly at this word it becomes clear that science wants to create knowledge. It is not meant that it already has knowledge but is looking for it. (Note by translator: Here is a game of words in German „Wissen schaffen", i.e. knowledge creating).

However, don`t let us be mislead: methods which include the non-rational and connect with the rational can offer solutions of undreamt volume and undreamt quality.

EXACTLY THIS COMBINATION OF RATIONAL AND NON-RATIONAL IS THE SOLUTION OF THE FUTURE.

And this is the base of Grigori Grabovoi`s teaching.

If we recognize and learn the essential, this approach becomes a blessing.

We need a **clear line into the depth** instead of getting bogged down into the breadth. The variety of the methods on the market shows the helplessness in these days and age.

Only the few genuine sources mostly offer depth in an issue: this is how we can find e.g. the real sources for the meditating ones:

• in the ancient Indian schools in the way they show themselves in the Veda and in the Baghava Gita
• in the Tibetan direction
• with Rudolf Steiner and his anthroposophy.

We have to search for a long time in the issue „physical, spiritual and mental health and excellent self-development" to find a genuine source which provides us with <u>undreamt of</u> levers.

• The Russians around Grigori Grabovoi are also such a genuine source and to this also contemporary.

Question: Where is the approach?

Answer: **Man isn`t a 3-dimensional creature but stands on the interface between life and the other world, between mind and soul on the one side and the physical body on the other side. Man connects these two worlds within himself.**

So if man connects mind, soul and matter within himself, then why shouldn`t he use methods which can exactly do that? These methods are justified just as scientifically as others. Only the ones who know a lot about that can judge it in the end.

Therefore: don`t let yourself be held back by people who are not able to judge this.

And: The genuine sources still have one thing in common: they offer depth and are usually appropriately hard to read.

Question: **Modern health methods come from America and Western Europe, but not from Russia. What can Russians then offer in such an issue?**
Answer: **At present, nobody is well-known in the world who at least is able to come up with the methods Grigori Grabovoi offers.**

Question: **What do we need God for?**

Answer: Everyone who ventures to real depth comes to God in the end. This was also valid for the great minds such as Max Planck who first became Atheists because of their research. The more deeply they did research the more they discovered God again. No really great (human) mind stayed stuck in the materialism and the rationalism.

Instead of calling God into question it is better to wonder whom it serves and what terrible price we have to pay for that we are being held tight in the material consideration and in the fun-society.

Who renders homage to e.g. the tennis God, soccer God, leisure God or money God, doesn`t only violate the 1st commandment but also then doesn`t have to be surprised if accidents, illness or impoverishment happen to him. There are clear connections and mechanisms which finally remove again the fun and the pleasant existence from us.

Question: What is this all good for me?

Answer: The number works of Grigori Grabovoi are a powerful help. Even more powerful this approach becomes combined with God, it is virtually based on it.

Rudolf Steiner has already predicted 100 years ago that Christ will appear again in the ethereal world. For everybody who knows the special manner of eyesight today, it is visible that Christ has already appeared and is active in the astral world.

> If we will learn again „to control constructively" instead of destroying egoistically, we also are able to get good help from the powerful side.

Question: How is e.g. modern medical knowledge being compatible with God?

Answer: God supports everything which serves the right further development and meets certain boundary conditions. There is further development in business life as well as in private or professional life and in recovery. **But the decisive question is whether our supposed further development is a development which runs in the right direction.**

Question: **And what is the right direction?**

Answer: Grigori Grabovoi has written about that in detail in his works and it also becomes clear in this book.

Question: **So what does Grigori Grabovoi mean with eternal development and eternal life?**

Answer: **This is very simple in the end: There are boundary conditions for all <u>appearances</u> of this world which have to be fulfilled so that something happens.** In our health endeavors, if we want to make use of the infinity (such as a mathematician does) for our lasting recovery, then we actually just need to understand how it works. Then it becomes very simple. The same applies to terms **like eternal development or eternal life.**

Related to eternity the so-called coincidences won`t become games of chance any more but they will become to what is planned to fall to us. This so-called positive coincidences can be increased. But whoever has only his advantage in mind will experience disappointments furthermore.

<u>Because:</u> **Everything we strive for has to be compatible with everything that all and everything others want. This is e.g. <u>one</u> of the boundary conditions.** If we observe the rules, then not only gates will be open to us but whole worlds.

> **If we satisfy all prerequisites, then our health plan becomes cont-rollable.** If we satisfy the above mentioned **boundary conditions**, then these **gates** also will get **open** for us.

Question: So what are the prerequisites for a successful recovery now?

Answer 1: There are 7 **essential prerequisites.** All of them have something to do with the spiritual-emotional attachment within us. The materialists may be bothered now that all of these 7 points **aren`t „hard facts".** They all should know that success comes virtually with the soft factors. Many scientists and businessmen of other branches already had to learn this lesson. **Not only faith moves mountains, the impulses of the soft factors can also do that.**

Answer 2: **The prerequisites are:**

1. Faith in God.
2. .. The appreciation of the functioning of love, harmony, luck and the joy of eternal development.
3. The ability to feel love and to be able to send love.
4. The understanding for the necessary change in us and in our life.
5. The will to control aim-orientedly.
6. Having patience (with himself) and humility.
7. Endurance and responsibility.

Question: And how shall this „esoteric gibberish" e.g. of the eternal development help me with my health?

Answer: As already told the recovery becomes much more controllable than we could imagine until now. **We have to be able to handle such im-**

pulses correctly. What was the understanding of „removing illness" until now is only one half of the wisdom.

> **If we consider e.g. the <u>eternal development</u> and bring our aim into line, then it can only arise from the correct control of <u>all</u> influencing factors. This would be so to speak the ideal case.**
> **<u>So one thing is clear:</u> If we satisfy all the conditions for this ideal case of eternal devlopment, then a shorter running recovery plan is on the ideal trace, of course.**
> **This is a mathematical law.**

Question: To the domain of cure:

Doesn`t every man has **the right to get help from above** (from the creator) anyway? I have been suffering already for month.

Answer: Whoever believes that **violates the commandment of humility.** As experience shows we have to pay arrogance expensively. **We are on the wrong way with arrogance.**

Question: **If I already have a big problem today, then I have to solve this one first. I need the help immediately. So how could it be that I do have to read for a long time first and maybe even change my character?**

Answer: With that we are getting to the **central point of the events.**

> Since thoughts and feelings form the 3-dimensional reality, every
> change within us influences the course of the earthly reality essenti-
> ally. Every recovery plan depends on the above mentioned soft fac-
> tors by those being involved in the plan.

Question: **If e.g. I am unlucky because of an accident or my knee both-
ers me, I have to look for it in the spiritual-emotional area?**

Answer: To look for can be a long lasting approach. **It is better and much
faster to free oneself from everything** that goes into the direction of ex-
cessive pride – egoism – vanity – domineering behaviour – lies – envy
– distrust – arrogance – hypocrisy – flattery – wrong sympathy – aggres-
sions – greed – miserliness – hate – weariness of life – malice - fanaticism
– despondence – mortification – self-abasement – doubt – stess - obstinacy
– irritability and much more other but not less dangerous qualities of the
human character.

This doesn't spare further-reaching searching but helps along at first.

Question: And how can I do that?
Answer: Grigori Grabovoi comments on that in his work „Unified system
of Knowledge" and Hugin Munin in the book „Practical Directory for the
‚Technologies and Methods of Grigori Grabovoi". **All of these negative
issues in man have to be solved.**

> *Question:* Do you claim that the resolution of such points positively influences all types of plans, that is a recovery plan or even a professional plan?
>
> *Answer:* **Exactly that is the order of the universe. We called into action (or people close to us) the accidents, illnesses and failures that happen to us by ourselves. Wrong thinking, wrong wanting, wrong feeling and wrong acting are the causes of our failures. And this is exactly why the key for solution is in the issues such as love, harmony etc.**

Question: Why should my professional failure or my lacking recovery depend on such wrong personality qualities (wrong thinking etc.), when the medicine provides all conceivable drugs?

Answer: **Man gets failures to think about it and to take another direction within <u>himself</u>. Nowadays most people experience God only rudimentarily.** If we recognized the cosmic truth, we would get to other behaviours and other successes. Whoever puts other gods above God doesn`t satisfy one of the prerequisites.

Question: If somebody harms me physically, financially or professionally, then the cause is obvious. What does this have to do with my wrong thinking, wrong wanting, wrong feeling etc.?

Answer: This looks quite different from the view of the universe.

> Negative things (thought, will, feeling, action) disrupts the harmonious development of the total system „universe". These deformations threaten to lead the total system into instability. Accordingly the universe starts countermeasures.

<u>Thus:</u> If we e.g. argue professionally or privately or are only agressive, we will get in form of countermeasures e.g. maybe physical failures or an unpleasant experience within our environment, that is in a completely different area. We will get paralyzed systematically. The countermeasures will get harder, if we aren`t reasonable. Almost each of us knows such cases of our environment, where everything threatens to break down or already is breaking.

But: Do not understand this harmony thinking wrong:Harmony thinking mustn`t lead to a wrong softness. The getaway into softness is used with pleasure for not taking the responsibility. If softness turns into a threatening or entered damage, because the misbehaviour was not demonstrated clearly (without getting agressive), then the other also can`t recognize his misbehaviour correctly. With that we do a disservice to society development and also to creation.

Question: The whole universe does move because of a trifle, does it?

Answer: The universe intervenes in everything that disturbs the **fine** structures of the universe.
<u>Because:</u> The more subtle the perturbed level, the greater the disorder.
<u>**AND:**</u> God decides whether something is a trifle. **Whoever believes to determine the standard by himself, collides with the law of humility.**

Question: So if I am a fighter , then I disrupt the order of the universe?

> *Answer:* **The way of thinking in the modern world has the drafts of a cancerous growth. Accordingly you can see what comes back to us by cancerous aspects in the body, in the professional as well as in the social and economic environment.**

Question: Where is the sense in that then?

Answer: The sense is to preserve the stability of the total system by „sections being switching off" which are no longer controllable.

Question: I am switched off?

Answer: The spreading of the destruction program is prevented by painful measures in the end. **Who doesn`t become reasonable at all, can only be stopped in the end by an early death or financial ruin.**

Question: Who in universe is disturbed by such a minor thing like e.g. „my desire to eat"?

> *Answer:* Again: What every single one wants is always clear. But **firstly** God decides whether something is minor or not and secondly the universe wants love, harmonious conditions, further development instead of destruction etc.
> **If we respect the prerequisites, then we will get everything. It may be funny to eat good food etc., but becomes dangerous and the wrong way, if it turns into an essential orientation. What was the 1st commanment again?**

Question: So I shall fight for harmony in the world?

Answer: A fight with others for harmony is paradoxical.

> **To reach a harmonious condition based on the unity with God by controlling is more promising than every fight.**

The amputated leg of an aggressive motorcyclist or the flop of a business-man by wrong competition are examples of a high price for a fight.

> **To offer attractiveness and to prepare oneself for an effort-saving, long-term effect are completely different qualities. It is about developing wholesome qualities.** Plans designed for harmony don`t disturb other people and creatures of the universe. Harmonious thoughts also don`t disturb the organization of the physical body of man.

Question: Why do so many things go wrong although people often try so hard?

Answer: **Purely externally regarded, this may look like that. But how could we know what is going on inside the supposedly unlucky person? Usually the faith of having done everything doesn`t reach far enough.** If we don`t care for our inner (mental-spiritual) growth, **then our recovery plan will run somehow, but not as successful as it could.** Here the key is in the overcoming of our ego.

Question: What is the difficulty?

Answer: **We know what the difficulties in our plans are and we have enough possibilities to find it out. For that it won`t fail. This is also valid for the emotionally and mentally weak points <u>within us</u>. But? There is** no but. The emotional-mental, weak points which altoghether cause destruction in us humans are traceable in many ways. But the lasting solution and the necessary change within us work only with the right turning to God in the end and the compliance with the prerequisites. And only the clairvoyant is able to see whether something really is dissolved. If we aren't able to see clairvoyantly, then we are only able to recognize or feel the effect of a change within us.

Although there are many people who believe to have already dissolved all negative influences within themselves with the common methods. But mostly it is a fallacy. Only the simple problematic cases can –maybe- be solved with the common methods. Only the acid test combined with God and a qualified clairvoyant will reveal the truth. **The demonstrating of a problem area isn't a solution yet.** Many methods mix there something up. Difficult cases can only be solved with God. Read what Grigori Grabovoi says to that.

Question: What to do?

Answer: To dissolve the negative influences **verifiably** and then to control e.g. by numbers.

Question: **And this is valid for the physical and also for the business plans? It is far too esoteric from the scientifical point of view.**

Answer: There is nothing esoteric with that. „Esoteric" means „secret teaching". **With the method of Grabovoi we just have much more and also very different control factors:** hard and soft. Whoever knows these connections will win. **This is a knowledge available for everybody today and not a secret teaching.** These control mechanisms are the same for private as well as business plans.

> Every plan has **material** influences (money, resources etc.), **psychological / personal** influences (characters of the involved ones etc.) and **influences determined by the situation / system** (universal control numbers). The universe is a system which not only offers control but also has a Creator.

Question: And how can we work with these soft factors?

Answer: There are clear step sequences for it. Now we are getting to the „pre-considerations" in the next chapter as a start.

1. PRE-CONSIDERATIONS

1.1 How numbers work

(Read to this Hugin Munin „Practical Directory for the Technologies and Methods of Grigori Grabovoi".)

a. Basis is the understanding of the construction of the universe.

b. Everything in universe is part of the Creator. The Creator is the actual reality.

c. God plays a part in everything.

d. The work foundation <u>below</u> God contains the <u>principles</u> for everything that comes to a realization at the levels under it. These principles are based on the realization techniques/ methods.

e. Principles are for example:

- the principle *bright/dark*
- the principle *active/passive*
- the principle *movement*
- the principle *energizing*
- the principle *control mechanisms*

f. These principles show that there is an infrastructure. The infrastructure needs an effect principle behind it with which it can work.

g. The effect principle exists in form of the *tree of life* which is contained in the *flower of life*. This 4-layered tree of life is a universal hologram.

h. This 4-layerness contains the reflection of the respectively higher level in the ones that are lying beneath. (spiritual level, mental level, astral level → rough materialed level)

i. The ubiquitous <u>information field</u> penetrates all 4 levels and with that every object and every event of the universe.

j. <u>Information</u> is put at the topmost level (= prototypes/templates). This information has contents and form (= geometry). **The decisive is the form.**

k. The energy fields lead to active information (in-form-ation).

l. If the form is being energized, then processes arise. Processes already are running at the astral level.

m. Typical appearances of energized information: Aura, color vision of a clairvoyant, feeling of vibrations in a part of the body or around it.

n. For our understanding **the decisively new** is not the information as a basis which then becomes energized, but the **geometric form of the information**.

o. **Energized forms of information at the astral level have an effect on the rough materialed world. They may not be mixed up with the energetic appearances of the 3-dimensional, material world (such as e.g. electricity).**

p. Since the hologram principle of the 4 different levels is valid everywhere, we also have very different control systems in the empire of the son.

q. **The control systems control the whole universe, all processes and all objects.**

r. God uses among others geometries:
- pyramids
- spheres etc.

s. Man, animals, plants and minerals aren`t purely earthly appearances, but lie on the interface between life and the other world.

t. **Man has conscious access to his control systems and to the control** systems for animals etc.

u. <u>Number sequences</u> are part of the geometric control systems.

v. - The control by numbers makes it possible to <u>influence</u> the own <u>health</u> and also life <u>circumstances</u>.

- If we use the number sequence we influence the <u>preparation</u> of situations at the astral level with that.

- And in the earthly world desired events arise accordingly, e.g. <u>recovery</u> events.

w. There is a geometric form in the information room for <u>every</u> process behind which there is a <u>basic</u> number sequence. Any basic number sequence can also be controlled/optimized by another number sequence.

x. The control by numbers is very advantageous, because:
- it is easy to handle
- it is precise
- it works even, if we are not able to see clairvoyantly.

y. What effect does the control have based on the eternal life? **How** could we **recognize** these **influencing of situations**?

Answer: **The situation structure changes.**

Example 1: **Increased so-called happy chances.**

Example 2: **Stable situations** (maybe e.g. quarrelsome neighbours move out…)

Example 3: **People who freezed us off earlier now contact us increasingly.**

Example 4: **Typical stumbling blocks disappear „as if by magic".**

Example 5: **Ideas are given to us, e.g. for a private change.**

Example 6: **We receive information, e.g. about a professional change, which offer us immediately new chances.**

Example 7: **The right thought comes at the right time.**

Thus: **Numbers are educational elements. Numbers form something. And so it goes without saying that it is our own interest to catch <u>as many</u> influencing factors <u>as possible</u>. In terms of eternity all coincidences are just events that we are able to control by logic.**

z. The **optimization** of the factors occupies a huge room.

Question: **Isn`t it better to control in advance the later upcoming bottleneck which we aren`t able to see today yet, so that everything is optimal later?**

Answer: **At every deviation of the norm put in concept (for eternal development) the sub-processes of our efforts are influenced in a way that we can stay on the way to eternal development.** The influencing from the part of the numbers is carried out here by the **right** thoughts at the **right** time or by necessary knowledge influx at the right time etc.

Thus: - With this method the otherwise usual intuitive thinking turns into system thinking, i.e. into exact thinking.

- If we are able to see the <u>spiritual</u> light with the 3rd eye, we will understand the according processes of the universe even more easily. We recognize that we have turned into creator. We also can understand that without seeing.

Welfare noticed: We have turned into creator but we are <u>not</u> God. Please don`t forget humility.

- If we aren`t clairvoyant, naturally we also create. But we first have to trust that everything goes its systematic way. Later we see the result (e.g. the recovery) in the earthly world.

2. PRELIMINARY NOTES

2.1. The classic Consideration to the Approach

Please list the steps that lead to cure in your opinion:

- Balanced meal?
- Dietary supplement?
- Body Exercise? Etc.

_____

_____

_____

2.2. The mental Order and its Importance

• The list of typical answers for the task in chapter 2.1 is known to you and us. We will refrain from the discussion about the classic answers.

• The variety of approaches and the variety of methods and means is very remarkable in connection with this. That should make suspicious. **As already mentioned in the preface – the „fragmentation" of an issue leads us away from the essential.**

• The area of spiritual cure is also threatened by this danger:

Question: Where do I start? Shall I direct my spirit to the body part or to the emotional situation? Do I take a number or a geometry?

• **It is important that you experience an improvement.**

• **The best way to achieve the aim is to make use of a <u>scheme</u>.**

<u>Because:</u> a) Then we will have a step sequence and won`t forget the one or other step.

b) In addition, we won`t overlook the one or other boundary condition, e.g. the creating of a unity with God by special key words.

c) We will save time because these always same steps will lead to an increase in speed.

• **<u>But:</u> Please don`t sink into <u>thoughtless</u> murmuring, just to save**

time by that. You don't do yourself a favor with that.

• Why do you think mantras and prayers are repeated over and over again? We become more and more conscious about the spiritual incantation. It's not sufficient to know the content only. We get from knowledge to emotional realization by the multitude of repetitions.

• The guide structure in the next chapter is not compulsory, but it is preferably used by those persons being already practiced. There are abbreviations very frequently in life. However, these **abbreviations** will **help** only **those who are well versed in their methods..**

If we strive for recovery, we mustn't take abbreviations which lead to a dead end in the end and which have stolen important time.

• **Question:** Can't I just take a number? That should suffice, shouldn't it?

Answer: You can't destroy anything with a number, since it works harmonizing.

<u>But:</u> Experience teaches that a number can help or also not. This is not due to the number but due to that we overlooked other boundary conditions.

• **Question:** Isn't it sufficient just to look at the graphic such as you can see in the books of Svetlana Smirnova?

Answer: We should know these graphics, since they support our imagination. Beyond that the graphics and the step sequences belong together.

Please read once more the above-mentioned points a) – c). Finally we have two parts of brain and both we have to use.

2.3. What do I do, if...

2.3.1 The recent <u>Beginner</u>

• **The recent beginner should take care to avoid to take any abbreviation way. If he nevertheless tries this, then he doesn`t have to be suprised if he won`t have any progress.**

To have a spiritual guide-line has proved itself for millenia. Please read to this again chapter 2.2.

2.3.2 The already <u>Practiced</u> (with Exercises)

• Many have practiced these methods already for years.

• **If there is no progress, then the indivual should examine in every layer of the guide- line whether he really takes everything into account.**

• The observation shows that there are stumbling blocks which mean the end of the way in a lot of cases. The **first** big **stumbling block** is e.g. that the fulfillment of the prerequisites is taken too lightly.

CONCLUSION: You can visit the greatest healers of this world for years, at best there will be a stop of the degeneration but no further healing.

BECAUSE: Each of the 7 prerequisites for the healing is very important (see chapter 4 later).

According to the observation, especially the mentally well trained make the greatest mistakes. The situation is not less dramatic with those who think they are spiritual or esoteric.

• **Stumbling block no. 2** is the confusion within the issue of the clear truthful order of the universe. Esoteric enthusiasm doesn`t really help (or even partly harms seriously). And the confusion of cause and effect then leads to the fact that we still do not get a toothache in connection with the spiritual cause which e.g. could be the result of a dispute around a property with the ex-partner.

• **Stumbling block no. 3 is the elimination of the phase of the controlled entry.**

• **Stumbling block** no. 4 is the cleaning phase. There`s less further progression without expert dissolution of negative information. Why often don`t help all these psychological setting-ups?

• **Stumbling block no. 5 provides a consistent line.**

With the help of a clairvoyant you are able to gain clarity more easily and control more specifically. But for that you need a good one. The ideal combination is a healer plus a clairvoyant. It is ideal (even for a given clairvoyance) when you control permanently.

Without the help of the above mentioned **healer and clairvoyant** you will have no choice but **to control permanently**. Who doesn`t do that and thinks to get to success with the least amount of effort is mistaken very much.

Such cases where the externally visible things of the body can be dissolved with little effort are encouraging. But are we then also already healed inside? **Or when will the problem return? It is better for everyone to go the way of <u>permanent</u> control, such as Grigori Grabovoi proposes.**

• **Who takes a NEW way <u>inside</u> will find the way back out of the valley.**

2.3.3 If nothing changes

• <u>On the one hand</u> there are changes which are <u>not</u> visible or don`t become visible immediately to the outside in the earthly world.
Every process runs at first at the mental, then at the astral and only then at the gross material level. Every measure causes something. The question is when will we see a reaction in the earthly world.

• Furthermore there are exercises that need an impulse so that the process starts to run. If it isn`t duly set up, then nothing will happen.

• Moreover, a negative information massiveness could hinder any efforts.

• And when we haven`t started correctly, this could also cause that nothing will happen. Usually then the key words for the right initialization are missing.

• **How you have to act correctly you will find in this book.**

• **Question:** So do you practice enough? Why should something change, if we don`t practice enough, i.e. if we don`t want to control.

• <u>On the other hand,</u> Grigori Grabovoi emphasizes over and over again that we should use as many different methods as possible. The reason for that is not only in the different efficiency factors, but also that we should get to know all the different methods.

2.3.4 The difference „simple case ←—→ complex case"

• **Complex cases can`t be cleared with means that are intended for the simple cases.** Read to that in chapter 4.6.6.2 „The complexity in an apparently simple issue".

2.3.5 When we don`t know exactly any more what to do.

• Then please look first at chapter 3.1 and then in chapter 3.2. There is an overview of the phases.

2.3.6 If I don`t have the time to practice in the period of 8 p.m. - 9 p.m. German time.

• 8 p.m. corresponds 10 p.m. Moscow time. The time can be transformed. „I transform the time of person „XY" to the time of 10 p.m. Moscow time." Please do this transformation with the exercises that are relevant to time after a clear entry before the respective exercise.

• The frequently heard idea that with 10 p.m. the Moscow time is meant, is not right. With 10 p.m. is always meant the time of the respective region, so for Germans in Germany the CET (= 10 p.m. wintertime).

2.3.7 If I can`t imagine anything.

• There is usually a misunderstanding here. Most think, they should be able to see something. But the abstract idea already suffices: just as like as we would see a vase and then close our eyes.

2.3.8 If I´m not able to concentrate enough.

• This is already a critical condition. The more important Grabovoi`s methods are.
• Check the methods for the psycho issues and the methods for the acquirement of new abilities.

2.3.9 If the offered <u>alternatives are too numerous</u> for me.

• The example of the cleaning methods shows that the methods have different results. Start with the alternative which is most useful for you or which you like the most.

2.3.10 If I don`t know how I can place the <u>numbers</u>.

• In this here available book are enough examples for that.

• Further information is available at Grigori Grabovoi 14) + 15) + 16) + 26)

2.3.11 What do I do, if I can`t remember the step sequences?

• **The technique of Grabovoi is based on concentration and not on meditation.** I.e. you can also **read** the step sequences. But please step by step and not according to the modern motto: „Yes, I already know. I don`t even need to read it.“

2.3.12 What do I do, if I don`t get down to infinity?

• Please imagine a railroad track. For the earthly observer the tracks lead **to a point** in the infinite distance. This is a step which may not be left out. If you cut out this step, then please don`t be surprised that the things arranged by you don`t make a lasting impression.

2.3.13 If I don`t know how I can give an impulse.
• We give the impulse e.g. by briefly thinking about the respective finger and conduct by a short breathing push through this finger. **There are processes which <u>don`t</u> start to run without an impulse.**

2.3.14 If I don`t like step sequences and prefer to work out of intuition.

• Intuition is good and can`t be big enough. Please read again the said to chapter 2.2. If you then still quarrel with the step sequences, then please realize that it is not about a forced discipline. It is virtually about **<u>self</u>-discipline** which leads us to success. If you then still quarrel, you should check whether you aren`t a victim of your arrogance.

2.3.15 If I can`t imagine the macro-level.

• Then please read Svetlana Smirnova1) or Grigori Grabovoi29). It is the area surrounding our 5 meter ball around us.

2.3.16 If I don`t feel the impulse of the heart.

• It is not about to perceive something from the heart, but to send an impulse of love which, as well known, comes from the area of the heart.

2.3.17 If I can`t feel love.

• Then it slowly becomes critical. In that case only studying and practicing helps. See 4.4.3.9. Maybe it also helps to beg God fervently to help us change our character. And for the change of character, there are several methods in this book.

2.3.18. If I can`t read well.

• Then in any case you can help yourself with the pictures of this book.

2.3.19 If my whole environment thinks that these exercises and the whole opinion behind it is „humbug".

• Then you have a serious problem. The minimum what you should do then immediately is an exercise for the harmonization of the family background. There are several possibilities to do that, among others also a number.

2.3.20 If I want to combine all these exercises with my daily mediation.

• The exercises of Grigori Grabovoi are based on concentration, not on meditation. It is good, if we take the physical attitude of meditation. Instead of trying to achieve the condition of inner emptiness, here it is about to go through a sequence of concentration exercises. The effect then comes to mind, body soul and consciousness. The „getting calm" plus concentration exercises is an excellent basis for your successes and your getting further. There also are exercises with which you are able e.g. to place new principles for changed behaviors.

2.3.21 If I like to listen to music for my sedation.

• Here the question comes up which music we are listening to. Whoever e.g. listens to „Requiem" by Mozart doesn`t have to be surprised when darkness arises.

2.3.22 If I`m afraid of cancer affected areas of others.

• Fear is not a harmonious feeling and thereby destructive. An aversion to something is as disastrous as sympathy for something. If we remain neutral, then we have broken our ties to this issue and our second chakra will get free from these bonds.

Indeed: Please don`t mentally intervene just like that in the morbid event. We should know exactly how we have to protect ourselves and how to handle this issue.

2.3.23 If I don`t know for how long I have to practice.

• According to Grigori Grabovoi we are able to pratice analogously to our feeling. However, who is practicing more than one hour a day, achieves a good progress according to experience.

2.3.24 If I don`t know what it is to canonize.

• To canonize means to secure the achieved, improved condition as a new starting point.

3. THE GUIDE STRUCTURE

3.1 The 9 Phases of the Guide Structure

Phase No.	Short term	Term	Aim
1	**PRE**	Pre-phase	Preparation + examination
2	**ENT**	Entry phase	- Synchronization with God - Fullfillment of the boundary conditions
3	**FOC**	Focusing phase	
4	**CLE**	Cleaning phase	
5	**DIA**	Diagnosis phase	
6	**RES**	Restoration phase	Rescue, raising
7	**SEC**	Securing phase	Sustainability
8	**EXI**	Exit phase	
9	**AFT**	The after-phase	To watch aftereffects

<u>Notes:</u>

a) We identify 9 essential steps for a session.

b) <u>Important:</u> The pre-phase may not be skipped. Even if we think to know it. At a short check of **the 7 points of this pre-phase** we may recognize that we are violating one of these points just right now again. **Who is in a hurry forgets e.g. humility „sometimes".** Who skips the „pre-phase" – no matter for what reason – makes a fast mistake which affects the success.

c) To have a **grid** for daily work makes the procedure easier.

d) The **always same way to enter and exit** saves you time and increases your consciousness at the same time. A complete session always contains the 8+1 phases!

e) Theoretically you can define the **main steps** for the phases of cleaning and reconstruction by yourself. But it is advisable to take the suggested ones because they all are proven.

f) The number of steps looks so extensively only at the beginning.

g) **Everything** we arrange mentally will **happen** in case we entered and exited correctly, even if we can`t see it.

h) A clairvoyant sees what e.g. changes in the aura (as a result of the given instructions).

Thus: If you don`t have a clairvoyant near you, then it will happen nevertheless.

i) Experience shows that we better should give some instructions 2-fold (during one session, but deferred) so that we can achieve the desired effect.

j) It could happen that the overall picture looks positive, but is dark at a check of detail nevertheless. This phenomenon has its correctness, because the angle of view of a clairvoyant is different at a complete consideration and a detail consideration.

k) Therefore, the check of a pictorial knowledge is always useful. Let yourself be guided by your feelings whether you want to check or not. Alternatively you can ask „in the upper world" to what extent e.g. the cells of an organ are free of negative information or negative energies.

l) **And:** The more frequent the session is, the more increase in success comes up.

m) **BUT: Without love for the target person nothing works at all!**

n) **And: Humility attitude is ncessary. Arrogance in any form harms us. And arrogance towards God is almost foolhardiness.**

3.2. Overview of the Sub-Items in the respective Phases

Phase No.	Short term	Phases with Sub-Items	Chapter
1	**PRE**	**The pre-phase**	**4.1.**
	PRE1	To clear the prerequisites	4.1.1.
	PRE2	The specification of the aim	4.1.2.
	PRE3	The aids	4.1.3.
2	**ENT**	**The entry phase**	**4.2. + 4.2.1.**
	ENT1	To make a unity with God	4.2.2.
	ENT2	To create the „sacred room"	4.2.3.
3	**FOC**	**The focusing phase**	**4.3.**
	FOC1	The partial steps of the focusing	4.3.1.
4	**CLE**	**The cleaning phase**	**4.4. + 4.4.1.**
	CLE1	Overview of the alternatives	4.4.2.
	CLE2	The partial steps of the cleaning alternatives a) – m)	4.4.3.

5	**DIA**	**The diagnosis phase**	**4.5.** + 4.5.1.
	DIA1	Overview of the alternatives	4.5.2.
	DIA2	The partial steps of the diagnosis alternatives a) – e)	4.5.3.
6	**RES**	**The restoration phase**	**4.6.** + 4.6.1.
	RES1	Overview of the alternatives	4.6.2.
	RES2	The partial steps of the restoration **Part I:** Alternatives a) – y)	4.6.3.
	RES3	**Part II:** Alternatives to the control of events	4.6.4.
	RES4	**Part III:** Alternatives with special solutions	4.6.5.
	RES5	**Part IV:** Complex restoration	4.6.6.
7	**SEC**	**The securing phase**	**4.7.**
	SEC1	The partial steps of the securing phase (V1)	4.7.1.
	SEC2	The partial steps of the securing-phase (V2)	4.7.2.
8	**EXI**	**The exit phase**	**4.8.**
	EXI1	The partial steps of the exit phase	4.8.1.
9	**AFT**	**The after-phase**	**4.9.**
	AFT1	**The observation**	4.9.1.
	AFT2	The building of protection	4.9.2.

4. THE SINGLE STEPS

4.1. The Pre-phase (PRE)

4.1.1. To clear the Prerequisites (PRE1)

• Many people already have **experience with unusual methods** which are desribed as „**non-rational**" in contrast to „**rational**".

• To be successful in recovery, personal and professional development, the **following prerequisites** are the ideal basis:

1. 1. The faith in God

A day has 86.400 seconds. How often do you think of God and act in conformity with him? The modern person usually has many Gods: the money God, the sports God, the leisure God, the family God, the work God etc. This is a clear violation of the 1st commandment.

Besides the commandments we have **even further guidelines, such as the virtues, the mortal sins** etc. **Who wants to have the most powerful help, the help of God, can`t ignore God in his life at the same time.** Who doesn`t believe in God doesn`t have to be surprised, if he e.g. doesn`t recover.

The list of modern Gods could be continued as many as you like:

The „God of greed", the „God of envy", the „God of miserliness", the „God of television", the „God of talking about illnesses or about others", the „God of criticizing" etc.

Let`s just look at the greed. This can manifest itself when eating, at the game in the stock market, at ambition in sports, at the desire for vacation trips etc. The misconduct is visible even more detailed in the following examples:

* The craftsman has caused a damage and suggest a compromise to the customer for compensation. The customer says no and prefers to be in a legal battle for a larger compensation sum. And loses the process.

* The pensioneer gives a signal to the healer that he has no money to lower the price of the treatment already in advance. In the same conversation he mentions his involvement in the stock market. In addition, he was angy about his losses in the stock market.

* The ex-husband suggests in the context of property disputes to take over the property including debt to zero. The ex-wife refuses and calls for a fee of 25.000 Euros. In the context of the ongoing division of their auction she risks losing 85.000 Euros and to be in debt for the rest of her life. This example happened even though the woman was referred to the commandment of God. Was it greed or injured pride?

Question: What do the 3 examples have in common with recovery?

Answer: <u>Firstly,</u> there is a violation of the order of God. The mildest consequences from it are failures and losses.

<u>Secondly,</u> the aura of the liver of the 3 persons was respectively dark. If the liver is blocked, the cognitive faculty of man interrupts or is affected heavily. The gall of the stock market player was obstinately dark. The annoyance over the losses left its traces.

<u>Thirdly,</u> they all had considerable physical problems. These health problems are already the results of an advanced misconduct.

AND: In all 3 cases the inner thought world was in the foreground. **They have put their corresponding problems above the love of God.** According to this situation they could hardly get out of their carrousel of thoughts.

<u>Fourthly,</u> every of the 3 persons believed to hold a justifiable request. Besides the greed, this way of thinking often is based on a justice fanatism. This behaviour is also a violation of the 1st commandment. **Whoever thinks to be able to put his scale over the scale of God is on the wrong way.**

<u>Fifthly:</u> With all 3 persons a heavy darkness was visible (by a clairvoyant's look) in the aura at the examination of the respective relation of the person to the 1st commandment.

<u>Thus:</u> **Without the consideration of the 1st commandment and without dissolving of this darkness worked out over decades, every attempt of recovery will be not very promising.** At best only small physical problems will be solved. How to make the competent dissolving a success is described in the book later.

Please also read to this:

→"Selected Lectures" by Grigori Grabovoi
→"Methods of Healing through the Application of Consciousness" by Svetlana Smirnova und Sergey Jelezky
→"Practical Directory for the Technologies and Methods of Grigori Grabovoi" by Hugin Munin

2. The understanding of the function of love, harmony, luck and joy of the eternal development.

Grigori Grabovoi has written in detail about these necessary qualities in „Joy of the eternal development". **Harmony-thinking e.g. requires a certain attitude of mind in the direction of general public. If we help others, then we help ourselves. There is a difference whether we just want to have our own health or whether we are asking to get better so that we are able to offer a factual and emotional use to others. And the help for others may not be limited to earthly-material help. Also when helping it depends on the right help.**

It is important to learn and to learn again how to make the wordings correctly and why it is so important for ourselves. Who doesn`t want to develop this understanding doesn`t have to be surprised, if he doesn`t recover. Who is ill wants his health. This is clear. But what use has the general public and the universe of e.g. an emotionally ill person getting well physically? Let us be true, the health is granted to everyone. It is just about the Question: „What is the ill person able to offer to e.g. the general public so that the universe grants him support." It results from this that the universe is helping the single person, if he always thinks of the harmonious solution for the general public first and afterwards thinks of himself.

An example:

A really ill person with spinal column problems begs for help after he requested help already 19 times at another place. With the 19 telephone calls there was a complete telephone time of more than 2 days. He transferred „generously" 100 euros to this place for that. He now even wants to induce the new healer to come over to him to the 150 km far away place. The healer presented 3 alternative suggestions for the transport of the ill person to the healer, the ill person refused all of them.

The egoism of the ill person let all sensible suggestions fall through. The ill person wanted to „have" but did not cooperate in any place.

The spinal column problems are based on violations of God. Don`t his sufferings still suffice the ill person? A recovery here is only promising, if man changes his understanding of the world and of other people. How we can work on that we see in this here available book.

Please also read to this:

→"Selected Lectures" by Grigori Grabovoi
→"Practical Directory for the Technologies and Methods of Grigori Grabovoi" especially understanding key No. 6+8 by Hugin Munin

3.The ability to feel love and to send love.

We can learn this ability. For this we have to practice, practice, practice. If we have read Grigori Grabovoi correctly, then we know that love is able to heal even material damages e.g. of equipment. **Who isn`t really able to feel love doesn`t have to be surprised, if he doesn`t recover.**

Many people have lost this ability in the age of materialism. Example:

A dentist has intensively taken care of his mother. But she nevertheless desinherited him in favor of his sister. He couldn`t or didn`t want to get over it. The dentist didn`t have any money problem. He merely couldn`t digest this chunk which his mother had served him. He claimed of himself he coudn`t really feel love. And then he died of a pancreatic carcinoma.

In this book we can see how we learn to feel love and how to dissolve such a shock.

Furthermore, please read to this:

→"Practical Directory for the Technologies and Methods of Grigori Grabovoi" by Hugin Munin

4. The comprehension for the necessary change within us and our life.

Our situation of today (e.g. physical, professional, family, financial etc.) is mainly the result of our thoughts, our will, our emotions and our actions. If not from this life, then from the former life. We consequently don´t need to strive that the others may change. **Whoever isn´t satisfied with his situation has to cause changes <u>within himself</u> at first.**

We can lament illness, accident etc. or regard it as luck which shall make us reconsider the journey through life and to take another direction. In doing so the inner changes are usually more important than those in the outer life. And whoever thinks he has to change other people is manipulating and on the wrong way with that.

Who doesn´t want to change doesn´t have to be surprised if he doesn´t recover.

Examples:
The examples from „1. Faith in God" also are valid here. A further example to think about is a woman who feigned her family a pregnancy at the age of 57 years. As this illusion was dissolved by the obvious truth after 8,5 month,

nettle rash appeared which lead to an established skin cancer later.

Instead of changing ourselves and our way of thinking, we usually prefer to criticize others. **At first we would need a scale to be able to critize and to quibble. The scale is able to show us who or what is wrong. With conscientious examination, however, we get to the fact that there could be no reasonable earthly scale besides the scale of God.** Instead of critizing others we better should go the right way by ourselves and let God direct us. Who criticizes others restricts the free will of the other one. This is a violation of God's law.

Furthermore, read to this:

→"Selected Lectures" by Grigori Grabovoi
→"Practical Directory for the Technologies and Methods of Grigori Grabovoi" especially understanding key No. 5+6 by Hugin Munin
→"Number Sequences of psychological Standardization" by Grigori Grabovoi

5. The will to control aim-orientedly with persistence

It is important to understand the teaching of Grigori Grabovoi right. Then we realize that the steering wheel is in our hands. We control all events with our consciousness. This is a process from morning to night. This also means that we will not be deterred by other from our new way. And we need the persistence to stay on the way instead of changing the direction constantly. If we don`t control aim-orientedly and prefer to jump from one issue to the next one, then we don`t have to be surprised if we don`t recover.

And whoever just drifts without controlling **insistently** will compulsorily leave the right way.

Because: The amount of numerous distracting thoughts (unlike the controlling ones) doesn`t help with the recovery but leads to destruction.

Examples:

Whether we constantly change the doctor or learn new, completely different methods in more and more workshops, both doesn`t really advance us. Others always transfer this way of acting in new partners or to new jobs or professions.

According to observation this also doesn`t carry the things on. Success won`t arise from the permanent change of directions. Such a change is like the hunt for a phantom.

Further development leads to success and not this kind of change.

An ill person who thinks to practice 10 minutes a day will be enough is seriously mistaken. The day has 1.440 minutes. The 10 minutes aren`t in any healthy relationship to the available time. The problem is that our mind is not really controlling in terms of a good direction at the rest of the time (and these are 99,31%). At 10 minutes of daily exercise we control only 0,69% of the available time.

Even if we subtract 16 hours for sleep and work, then only a ridiculous 2,08% (!) of active controlling result from 10 minutes to 480 minutes (8 hours). **The rest of time we are following wrong Gods (97,92%).** And here it is already calculated very generously to our favor, because the working time and the bedtime can`t be classified really „neutral“. **We won`t get too far with a few times of „short“ practicing.**

If a method of control was given to us now, then we just will have to learn how and how often we have to control.

And for this it will be sufficient, if we have a good look at this method

of control more and more deeply. **If we study the here available book exactly, then we already get to a considerable depth.**

Furthermore, read to this:
→"Practical Directory for the Technologies and Methods of Grigori Grabovoi" especially understanding key No. 6+8 by Hugin Munin

6. To have patience (with yourself) and humility
Impatience is a sign of uneasiness and strain. This is a destructive condition. Harmony, however, always exudes calm. Peace of mind has nothing to do with passivity. God sets the clock, not we do. **If we demand something impatiently, it is a sign of arrogance towards God.**

If we don`t want to become humble, we don`t have to be surprised if we don`t recover. A certain impatience is understandable, but not helpful although, in case we have traveled the world for 20 years and visited the greatest healers.

Cure can`t be called in. Doubtful esoteric-approaches have brought this nonsensical thought into the world. Humility can be learned and gives patience. **We only can experience cure as a gift and support it by permanent right control. In this book it becomes obvious how extensively we are able to control.** These methods of control are already godsend. Now it is up to us to become active to the right direction and to patiently prepare ourselves for the results.

7. Persistence and responsibility
The more confident we are of our destination, the more persistent we are. Doubts about the accuracy of our way prevent our persistence on our way.

It is our job to control <u>constantly</u>. **This is an ongoing task for our life. Who does not control with persistence doesn`t have to be surprised, if he doesn`t recover.**

Examples:

It became unfashionable to practice. We can see the result in the young generation who even doesn`t master the simple multiplication.

And if the driving schools would do the same, then may be we would never be able to get our driver`s license.

It is part of our responsibility to help others. Grigori Grabovoi clarified this. If we master something new it is our duty to pass this knowledge also on to others. We can hardly help someone who likes to keep his advance of knowledge to himself, because with his arrogance he violates the laws of God again.

BUT IF WE MEET ALL THIS 7 REQUIREMENTS, THEN OUR RECOVERY-PLAN BECOMES CONTROLLABLE. AN ATTRACTIVE REWARD IS WAITING FOR US!

4.1.2 The Specification of the Aim (PRE2)

Who doesn`t set his aim exactly can`t arrive there either. **The statement „I want to get healthy" is e.g. no exact specification, if the person has <u>several</u> problems.**
To get the help of God it requires a little bit more precision.
An example: „The skin at the left foot" is something else than „The skin between the small toe and the toe neighbouring at the left foot".

<u>BUT:</u> We learn that in this book using many examples.

And the aim is e.g. „Restoration of the norm of the Creator for all cells of the skin between the left…". <u>Because:</u> The Creator has provided the norm.

In no way it is sufficient just to say „All cells of my body…".

4.1.3 The Aids (PRE3) / Time Axis, Time Transfer, Pictures

a) Grigori Grabovoi doesn`t provide material aids. He also has spoken about the influence of crystals. However, you can refer to him and read his books in a quiet moment. [18]

b) A <u>mental</u> aid is the **time axis** of Z- ∞ to Z+ ∞ for a person. The imagination of such a time axis in front of us which is going from left to right is sufficient. Z- ∞ is on the left of us, Z+ ∞ on the right. Sometimes it is very advisable to work with the time. Please read more about this time axis by Grigory Grabovoi. [17]

c) Another aid is the **silvery-white cube** which Grigori Grabovoi has installed for everyone. It absorbs the negative entities and transforms them to white, divine light. We can use it. We will find the graphic for that by Svetlana Smirnova. [1]

d) The **used time** can be handled differently. **We have several possibilities. Especially advantageous is the time 10 p.m. to 11 p.m. [6] It doesn`t matter where we experience this time since the functionality is established in the way that it is converted to the respective meridian. We have 3 possibilities:**

1) Transfer of the time for a person to 10 p.m. Moscow time (s. 4.6.3.3.).

2) To practice at 10 p.m. German time.

3) If we aren`t able to practice at 10 p.m., then we could transfer our time analogously to 4.6.3.3 into German time. Or also in accordance to 4.6.3.25.

e) **Contemplation on pictures:**

The effect is the same **like** e.g. **of the healing effects** in front **of an icon.** The effect of healing could happen when the painter was working in a very specific way. The effects can go up to miracles. We also can get in connection with the picture mentally without seeing it. All the pictures were proved positively in their effects by clairvoyants. For the effect of the pictures, the in chapter 2.3.3 said, is valid.

All of the 5 pictures in this book are from **Sergey Jelezky.** 37)

f) **The mental order:** Please read to this again chapter 2.2 and 4.1.1, point 2.

g) The **clairvoyance** is an aid. Read to this chapter 4.6.6.1.

4.2 The Entry Phase (ENT)
4.2.1 Notes to the Entry Phase

1) Like it is visible in the work „Joy of the eternal Development", **we need** certain **elements such as joy, luck etc.** so that we can reach the right mental level. These elements are taken into account in the wordings of „entry" and „exit".

2) Here it is about keywords which may not be just left out.

3) If you enter in the here suggested way you can be sure to reach the right

level. This way is proven sufficiently. With this way of entry we get to the **macro level** and furthermore to all levels.

4) The procedure of a healing session for us has to be done best in a **smooth, upright sitting position.** To seat is better than to lie down. And the feet should stand on the ground.

Please note that here it is only about the position and not about meditation. Grigori Grabovoi`s method is based on concentration and not on meditation.

5) If we work on another person, then he may lie in front of us.

4.2.2 The partial Steps of the Entry Phase: To make a Unity with God (ENT1):

Steps	Meaning	How to do?
E1		„I`m in spirit and full of humility.“
E2	To direct the spirit on to the soul.	„I enter my soul and take position at the point of archiving.“
E3	To accomplish an infinte action.	„I see and act like the Creator with his physical body of the uniform God sees and acts.“ + **To send the feeling of love**
E4	To set into the creative area:	881881881
E5	To go onto the macro level and to arrange for every creature.	„Macro-control, please.“

E6	Heart impulse with message	„Rescue and **harmonious** development for everyone + everything. Also for me, please." + to send **golden light** „Love at first for the Creator and then for everyone and everything else."
E7	Concentration/imagination 1	„I am in the eternal **lighting current of eternity + at all levels.**"
E8	Concentration/imagination 2	„I am the **infinite cosmos** and the **joy** of its **infinite, eternal** further development."
E9	Rescue symbol + impulse	Ray of **luck** + 4-leaved cloverleaf
E10		„Christ, please accompany this process."

Note 1: With **E1** the time has come to breathe as slowly as possible, but rhythmically in and out.

Note 2: In **E2** to concentrate the breath, impregnated with love, on breastbone-end (for entry) and to breath it out at this point. And to direct a part of the breath at the end through the right sole of foot into mother Earth.

Note 3: To form in a symbol the **standing and lying 8** in **E9** (like a 4-leaved cloverleaf).

Note 4: We mentally speak what is put into quotation marks. The therapist can also speak out loud these instructions.

Note 5: The sequence of numbers in **E4** helps with the development of the spiritual view.

Note 6: In **E6** there is a certain order which has to remain the same. Please read to this again chapter 4.1.1, point 2 „The understanding...".

Note 7: In **E6** we see in the second sentence our current of love to the Creator.

4.2.3 To create the „sacred Room" (ENT2):

Steps	Meaning	How to do?
E11		„**To cut** all connections to points with negative information or negative energy at the apartment border/ property border."
E12		„**Cleaning** of the whole area of the apartment/ the property with the wall of light of the Creator. And removal of all negative entities to the divine level for the turning into the light in the silvery-white cube."
E13		„Cleaning up to **the purity degree of the Creator.**"
E14		„Restoration of the **paradise character** of this apartment/ property with luck, joy of the eternal further development, with harmony and with love. First of all love for the Creator and then for everyone and everything else."

Note 1: In **E11** it is about the room in wich we are.

Note 2: To build the wall of light in **E12** mentally over the whole breadth of the room and while doing that to think about the imagination of the removal of negative entities.

4.3 The Focusing Phase (FOC)

4.3.1 The partial Steps of the Focusing (FOC1)

4.3.1.1 Alternative a): The focusing on a person

Steps	How?
F1	„I see the time axis from $Z - \infty$ to $Z + \infty$ of person XY.“
F2	„Concentration forefinger **on the left**“.
F3	„I place the number sequence 938179 and ask for the help of concentration.“
F4	„Light sphere, please.“
F5	„I load into these sphere … the aura of person „XY“ / the state of health of „XY‘.“
F6	„I ask for the presentation of all cells of the hypophysis.“

Note 1: Instead of „XY“ we can name ourselves or someone other.

Note 2: Please read to the approach of time axis Grigori Grabovoi in „System of the education“ [17] and in this book chapter 4.1.3.

Note 3: To think the light sphere in F4 directly in front of the left forefinger, 2mm away, diameter 2mm.

Note 4: The real focusing contains **F1-F5**!

Note 5: The clairvoyant sees e.g. a light area oder a light space.

Note 6: Non-clairvoyance is no problem!

Note 7: The focusing creates clearness and supports the concentration.

Note 8: This alternative a) is the normal case of proceeding.

Note 9: F6 is listed to give an idea how it e.g. could go on.

4.3.1.2 Alternative b) The focusing in special cases

Steps	How?
F7	„I see the time axis from $Z-\infty$ to $Z+\infty$ of person XY."
F8	„I place the number sequence 938179 and ask for the help of concentration."

Note 1: This alternative to 4.3.1.1 is needed only in certain cases.
You will see that in this book in the respective exercises later.

4.4 The Cleaning Phase (CLE): The Rescue from negative Pressures
4.4.1 Notes

There are negative appearances in the mental room **and** in the astral room.

• **If they are stuck in our aura, then we feel a malaise. Who is not able to see clairvoyantly, at least feels something or even pain.**

• These appearances are connected with our inside, with our personality strucutre.We attract the dark with our own wrong thoughts, wrong feelings, wrong will impulses and wrong actions. Since we „worked out" the largest portion of our present personality structure in earlier lives, we have to do something against the consistently upcoming darkness.

• If we do nothing, then illnesses will arise from it.

• If we work e.g. with numbers in the direction of recovery, then the nested dark entities within us try to defend themselves.

• There are **4 ways** to escape from this darkness. These ways are no alternatives, but all have to be gone.

a) Permanent control, i.e. to have a positive effect on us permanently.

<u>Because:</u> Every positively mental infuencing control is faster than a progressive illness. So the dark can not settle.

b) To change the character.
<u>Because:</u> We attract the dark by ourselves. A completely pure character can cross an atom contaminated room without harm..

c) To dissolve the dark, i.e. to clean the aura.

d) To ask God fervently to clean us.

• The perfect health is in our own hands, but can`t be reached without the right reference to God.

• The construction of a preventive protection only makes sense when we have cleaned up inwardly.

• Our well-being is always a question of „often-enough-cleaning-and-control".

• Since we are liing in this world full of activities, we will be polluted over and over again, too.

• It is clear that a preparatory cleaning is only one important step of the restoration.

4.4.2 Overview of the Alternatives of Cleaning (CLEI): A helpful Variety!

Alternative	Reinigung
a)	The basic cleaning
b)	The extended basic cleaning
c)	Three light columns with colored light
d)	By cylinder on the head
e)	Soul-ball on pyramid of the Creator
f)	By crystal of soul
g)	By sending love into the past, present and future
h)	To clean body fluids (blood, lymph,...) by cube-cone-cube
i)	Cleaning of the soul by cell of God/ love
j)	By light shower
k)	By harmonization of present
l)	By balls in front of root of the nose and on head
m)	Cleaning of the chakras by spheres
n)	Cleaning of consciousness
o)	Cleaning by connecting with nature

Note 1: The possibilities of the alternatives of the way of cleaning are numerous.

Note 2: If the entry (according to chapter 4.2) is completed cleanly, then according to observation <u>almost every</u> job for cleaning is executed.

Note 3: Sometimes the aura is bright again already after a basic cleaning.

Note 4: But experience shows that usually the combination of different types of cleaning leads to purity. An accompanying clairvoyant is an advantage, because we are able to see when we can stop.

Note 5: Experience shows that the combination of the alternatives

b) basic cleaning	+ e) soul-ball on pyramid	+ f) crystal of soul	+ i) cleaning by cell of God

usually brings a good result, on which also a non-clairvoyant can rely.

Note 6: In contrast, a rescue from a <u>negative</u> information massiveness can no longer be named as a cleaning, because such a massiveness causes significant deformation in the field structure around man. This is why this kind of dissolving takes place in the context of restoration **(see chapter 4.6)**. Please read to this Grigori Grabovoi. [8]

Note 7: Please also note that we have seperate procedures for the cleaning of soul and for consciousness.

4.4.3 The partial Steps of the Cleaning (CLE2) in 13 Alternatives

4.4.3.1 Alternative a): The <u>basic</u> cleaning

Steps	Cleaning
ENT	**Entry** like in example **ENT1 + ENT2**
FOC	**Focusing** like in example **FOC1 (F1-F5)**
CLE	**Cleaning steps:**
C1	„**To restore** all points of penetration **according to the norm of the Creator.**" [1]
C2	„**To restore** all cells of the hypophysis **according to the norm of the Creator.**"
C3	„**To restore** all cells of the thyroid gland **according to the norm of the Creator.**"
C4	„**To restore** all cells of the liver **according to the norm of the Creator.**"
C5	„**To restore** all cells of the central nervous system **according to the norm of the Creator.**"
C6	„**To restore** all cells of the peripheral nervous system **according to the norm of the Creator.**"
SEC	**Transmission:** like in **chapter 4.7.1.**
EXI	**Exit: like in chapter 4.8.**

Note 1: The basic cleaning is often <u>not</u> sufficient, but very important.

Note 2: Despite the many alternatives the basic cleaning should always be the first measure of cleaning.

Note 3: The clairvoyant sees how the cells get into movement more and more and brightness comes into the aura.

Note 4: If we leave the house, then we might catch something negative again.

Note 5: And if somebody comes near you, then already it is very difficult to protect yourself.

Note 6: A good approach is a repeated cleaning for a few times a day.

4.4.3.2 Alternative b): The <u>extended</u> basic cleaning

Steps	Cleaning
ENT	**Entry** like in example **ENT1 + ENT2**
FOC	**Focusing** like in example **FOC1 (F1-F5)**
CLE	**Cleaning steps:**
C1	„**To restore** all points of penetration **according to the norm of the Creator.**"
C2	„Please close the aura with devine light."
C3	„To clean all cells of the organism with holy water."
C4	„**To restore** all cells of the hypophysis **according to the norm of the Creator.**"
C5	„**To restore** all cells of the thyroid gland **according to the norm of the Creator.**"
C6	„**To restore** the thyroid-gland-**<u>control</u>** according to the norm of the Creator."
C7	„**To restore all connections of the body parts with each other to the norm of the Creator.**"
C8	„**To restore** all cells of the liver **according to the norm of the Creator.**"
C9	„**To restore** all cells of the central nervous system **according to the norm of the Creator.**"
C10	„**To restore** all cells of the peripheral nervous system **according to the norm of the Creator.**"
C11	„**To restore** all cells of the gastrointestinal tract **according to the norm of the Creator.**"
SEC	**Transmission:** like in **chapter 4.7.1.**
EXI	**Exit:** like in **chapter 4.8.**

Note 1: Read to **C6**: Chapter 10 of the work „Uniformed System of Knowledge" about the distorted impulses (= zigzag or lightnings). The impulses of the thyroid gland control a lot of processes. Therefore you should understand this exactly and also how the impulse is placed correctly.

Note 2: Experience shows that the control by the thyroid gland is disturbed in the case of many people. **If you set up this control over and over again, many problems will be superfluous.**

Note 3: Similar is with **C9**. But here you can help with the 4-ball-technology. You will find the graphic to this at Svetlana Smirnova. 1)

Note 4: The liver also should be worked on in addition. With the aim to ask Christ to take even the smallest negative entities to the divine level for the transportation into the light to the silvery-white cube.

Note 5: If you have left your protected area, e.g. the apartment and you have returned, this cleaning is usually necessary.

Question: Why?

Answer: Because the cognitive faculty of people can be blocked by the liver. The thought blockades are in the liver and not in the brain.

4.4.3.3 Alternative c): 3 light columns with <u>colored</u> light

Note 1: The methods, later described in chapter 4.6.5.2, are also suitable for cleaning purposes.

Note 2: By the contribution of our wish, we are able to escape here from a certain burden, e.g. arrogance.

Note 3: This exercise is much more powerful than it seems at first.

Note 4: The clairvoyant sees the light events.

Note 5: The cleaning also happens, even if we aren`t able to see any colors.

4.4.3.4.Alternative d): The deduction of negative thoughts by cylinder on the head[6]

Note 1: With that, we are able to deduct into blue sky negative thoughts and also negative cell information at the moment of their formation.

Caution: The cylinder must not overlap.

AND: One cylinder per concrete issue, there is no other way.

Question: Why is this measure important?

Answer: With that we **prevent** the formation of **next negative** cells.

Note 2: The clairvoyant sees not only the cylinder and the outgoing rays, but also e.g. how the aura is brightening step by step after the installation of the cylinder.

Note 3: A variation of this alternative is to Note the number „1888948" for the conversion of the negative into positive.

Thus: A negative information may not even arise at the thinking level. We derive two things by that:

a) Thoughts

b) (Negative) information for the cells

4.4.3.5.Alternative e) Soul-ball on pyramide of the Creator/ ozone

Steps	Cleaning
ENT	**Entry** like in example **ENT1 + ENT2**
FOC	**Focusing** like in example **FOC1 (F1-F5)**
CLE	**Cleaning steps:**
C1	„I see the pyramid of the Creator with the sphere of my soul on the top."
C2	„The pyramid is on the inside of the 5m sphere of the consciousness."
C3	„The light of the absolute comes out of the pyramid."
C4	„The pyramid opens a bit, receives my soul sphere and illuminates it."
C5	„The soul sphere starts to shine increasingly."
C6	If it is illuminated now, then the pyramid opens and my soul sphere glides into the pyramide."
C7	„At this moment reactive ozone which **transforms the content of my soul to the norm of the Creator** is released."
SEC	**Transmission:** like in **chapter 4.7.1.**
EXI	**Exit:** like in **chapter 4.8.**

Note 1: You will find the graphic to this exercise at Svetlana Smirnova. . 1)

Note 2: This exercise should always be done right after the basic cleaning.

Note 3: The clairvoyant sees how it gets **very bright all around.**

Note 4: This exercise should be part of the standard repertoire.

Note 5: This exercise supports the (re)structuring of the soul.

Note 6: The positive cleaning effect must not lead to the belief that all pressures of the past would be cleared up with that. Merely the „latest" pressures are cleared up with that.

4.4.3.6. Alternative f): To activate the crystal of the soul

Steps	Cleaning
ENT	**Entry** like in example **ENT1 + ENT2**
FOC	**Focusing** like in example **FOC1 (F1-F5)**
CLE	**Cleaning steps:**
C1	„I see the crystal of my soul."
C2	„I give an impulse on its vibration structure for its activation now."
C3	„The activation takes place in accordance with the standard measure of the Creator."
SEC	**Transmission:** like in **chapter 4.7.1.**
EXI	**Exit:** like in **chapter 4.8.**

Note 1: We increase our oscillation frequency with that and **surveyable** pollutions disappear.

Note 2: This exercise is suitable, if you feel tired.

Note 3: It is also interesting that the crystal still starts to shine even in aged people. This is an indication of vitality.

Note 4: The clairvoyant sees the crystal and how it brightens and then shines.

Note 5: The changes of the crystal are announced very widely, e.g. the tip of the crystal could multiply. Or one of the crystal „columns" gets much bigger.

Note 6: Of course the crystal of **other** people also becomes visible at a corresponding focusing.

Note 7: The „crystal of the soul", the „flower of the soul" and the „book of life" are part of the 3 important representations of man's soul condition. The way the crystal shines, the same way the flower blossoms out. And the „book of life" can be renovated correspondingly.

Note 8: It is particularly interesting that this „book of life" often appears as a picture to people who promise an essential change in their life towards God. Sometimes it even gets visible how the change is registered.

4.4.3.7. Alternative g): Cleaning by sending love to the past, presence and future

Steps	Cleaning
ENT	**Entry** like in example **ENT1 + ENT2**
FOC	**Focusing** like in example **FOC1 (F1-F5)**
CLE	**Cleaning steps:**
C1	„I´m now sending infinite love on the time axis **to the left** to the events of my past." + impulse
C2	– 20 seconds break –
C3	„Now I am sending love to all events of the present." + impulse
C4	– 20 seconds break –
C5	„Then I send endless love on the time axis **to the right** to my future." + impulse
SEC	**Transmission:** like in **chapter 4.7.1.**
EXI	**Exit:** like in **chapter 4.8.**

Note 1: The **impulse** is given for each of the **past** and the **present by the right forefinger.** And for the **future by the right little finger.**

Note 2: In **C3** we send straight forward.

Note 3: The clairvoyant sees the meandering light worm that goes into the past and future.

Note 4: Since every wrong thought, every wrong feeling, every wrong will impulse and every wrong action start their own way to the future, we have placed in all our lives a huge number of wrong impulses which we cannot survey.

Note 5: Due to the fact that each of our thoughts, feelings etc. have gone their own way since primeval times and many incarnations, a wide network results from that we should clean with infinitely great love.

Note 6: However, the removal of negative information massiveness is not yet achievable with that.

Note 7: With this method you can place the number sequences for harmonization of the past, present and future at the same time. You will find the numbers at Svetlana Smirnova 1). For the placing of the numbers, please comply e.g. alternative b) in chapter 4.6.3.

Note 8: To the effect of the numbers, please also read chapter 4.4.3.11.

4.4.3.8. Alternative h): Cleaning of body fluids

Steps	Cleaning
ENT	**Entry** like in example **ENT1 + ENT2**
FOC	**Focusing** like in example **FOC1 (F1-F5)**
CLE	**Cleaning steps:**
C1	„I introduce the structure „cube-in cone-in cube" **in the aorta, about 10 cm <u>atfer</u> the cardiac output** of a person XY."
C2	„Cleaning of all toxins, pollution and contamination of organic and inorganic type."
C3	„Restoration of all cells of the blood to the norm of the Creator."
C4	„I place the number sequence **1843214** into a light-sphere with golden light."
C5	„And place the light-sphere into the structure „cube-cone-cube."
SEC	**Transmission:** like in **chapter 4.7.1.**
EXI	**Exit:** like in **chapter 4.8.**

Note 1: It is about 3 geometries which are nested into each other.

Note 2: The structure should **not** be placed **too close to the heart**. This came as a clear instruction from „above".

Note 3: This cleaning can be used for blood, lymph, the hormone system, isolated organs or cells.

Note 4: We are here at the standard of cleaning. Please compare with alternative „w" in chapter 4.6.3 "Alternatives of the restoration".

Note 5: This example here refers to blood. Of course another sequence of numbers has to be used in **C4** at another body fluid.

Note 6: The clairvoyant sees how the blood brightens very fast and he also sees the activity e.g. of the blood cells.

Note 7: If an illness is already in the blood, then hurry is advisable. According to Rudolf Steiner the systems of the organism are designed to do everything to protect the blood as the central system of man from degeneration.

Note 8: The cleaning of blood from contamination could improve the vitality.

4.4.3.9 Alternative i): Cleaning of the soul by the cell of God/ love (= space of the creative love)

Steps	Cleaning
ENT	**Entry** like in example **ENT1 + ENT2**
FOC	**Focusing** like in example **FOC1 (F1-F5)**
CLE	**Cleaning steps:**
C1	„„I try to get in touch with the cell of God below the left shoulder-blade.“
C2	"I imagine how the flow of divine love streams into me at this place and draw this flow towards me."
C3	"I can feel how this flow of divine love fulfills me increasingly. + I give an impulse to the uvula in the throat."
C4	"**I intensify** this love within myself. A fullness forms.“
C5	"I **connect** the flow with **the cells** that are close to the cell of God (within me) now."
C6	„„I can feel how these cells are also <u>surrounded</u> by the same love which fulfills me.“
C7	"I spread this love **into** all these cells now."
C8	"I give the impulse now 'spreading of love on all cells of my body'.“
C9	"I can feel how the whole body fills with love."
C10	"If the love is intensified within my body now, then I let this love stream out from under my chest to the outer world."
C11	**"The love flows into me now, through me and out of me again."**
C12	"In this condition I can feel the answer-love of other people and the world."
SEC	**Transmission:** like in **chapter 4.7.1.**
EXI	**Exit:** like in **chapter 4.8.**

Note 1: Since love is the greatest power in the universe, we can't repeat this exercise often enough. **A method with a very powerful effect.**

Note 2: The rescuer cell appears often. And the clairvoyant sees how the rays of love flow into the body, how they are condensed into golden light etc. and finally stream to the outside. Light spheres also like to form a flower at the end. Christ becomes visible more often.

Note 3: The impulse opens the room and the love streams. The love removes negative information.

4.4.3.10. Alternative j): Cleaning by light shower

Steps	Cleaning
ENT	**Entry** like in example **ENT1 + ENT2**
FOC	**Focusing** like in example **FOC1 (F1-F5)**
CLE	**Cleaning steps:**
C1	„I go and stand in the light current of the Creator."
C2	„Cleaning with holy water please for all cells of my physical, astral and mental body."
SEC	**Transmission:** like in **chapter 4.7.1.**
SEC	**Exit:** like in **chapter 4.8.**

Note 1: With that we are cleaned from all negative information (= mental level) and all negative energies (= astral level). Though the process then takes its time and the clairvoyant often sees no longer differentiatedly. The in alternative d) in note 4 said is also valid here.

Note 2: The clairvoyant sees cleaning violet light.

4.4.3.11 Alternative k): Cleaning by harmonization of the <u>present</u>

Note 1: The cleaning with number **71042** harmonizes the present.

Note 2: No matter what you are planning, the ideal time for this harmonizing cleaning is directly before it. It is a must for everyone who wants to help others.

Note 3: The clairvoyant sees how e.g. a broad river of brightness arises at the clearing up of the present.

Note 4: If we work with the number of the harmonization of the past, then you can see how this change of past causes a movement in the future. Among others a ball could move itself on the time axis at the future part or the Akasha finger of the right hand could announce a change. To get the results in present and future from the events corrected in the past there is a number in the book „Numbers for a successful Business". And at the change of future by number sequence e.g. flowers, butterflies or a basket full of eggs appear. Man blossoms out, transforms himself etc.

4.4.3.12 Alternative l): Cleaning by balls in front of the root of the nose and on the head

Note 1: This exercise is described very well- also graphically- in the literature of SVET-Centre. 12)

Note 2: This exercise is suitable in case you are tangled in a thought which doesn`t let you go any more.

Note 3: A problem, e.g. also a thought which don't let us go, is stuck in front of the nose and handicaps both the free mind and the 3rd eye.

Note 4: Don`t make the problem of the other one to your own.

4.4.3.13 Alternative m): Cleaning of the chakras by spheres

Steps	Cleaning
ENT	**Entry** like in example **ENT1 + ENT2**
FOC	**Focusing** like in example **FOC1 (F1-F5)**
CLE	**Cleaning steps:**
C1	„Light sphere in front of the right forefinger, please."
C2	„I load this sphere with golden light, with love, with harmony, with luck and with the joy of the eternal further development." + impulse
C3	„A copy of this sphere please around the **root chakra. Transfer.**" + impulse
C4	„Another copy around the **sacrum chakra**. Transfer." + impulse
C5	„Another copy around the **solar plexus chakra**. Transfer." + impulse
C6	„Another copy around the **life energy chakra**. Transfer." + impulse
C7	„Another copy around the **throat chakra**. Transfer." + impulse
C8	„Another copy around the **chakra of the 3rd eye**. Transfer." + impulse
C9	„Another copy around the **crown chakra**. Transfer." + impulse
C10	„Light connection with white light from the hypophysis to each of the set spheres."
C11	„Please restore the mental matrix and the astral matrix **to the norm of the Creator**."
SEC	**Transmission:** like in **chapter 4.7.2.**
EXI	**Exit:** like in **chapter 4.8.**

Note 1: The chakras and matrices are „relay stations" for information and life energy and have to be cleaned ideally once a week.

Note 2: The clairvoyant sees the spheres, how the chakras are getting brighter and how they start to move again.

Note 3: The negative information <u>massiveness can`t</u> be dissolved with that excercise either, but has to be worked on by restoration.

Note 4: We have to keep in mind here that the securing runs differently than in chapter 4.7.1, which describes the most frequent way of securing. The difference arises, because in this case we come from the right forefinger.

4.4.3.14 Alternative n): Cleaning of the consciousness

Steps	Cleaning
ENT	**Entry** like in example **ENT1 + ENT2**
FOC	**Focusing** like in example **FOC1 (F1-F5)**
CLE	**Cleaning steps:**
C1	„I take a divinely pure screen to my hand."
C2	„I place this divinely pure screen in front of eve-ry **screen and** every **mirror of my consciousness** now."
C3	„This screen shall lead all screens and mirrors to divine purity and establish the norm of the Creator within me."
SEC	**Transmission:** like in **chapter 4.7.1.**
EXI	**Exit:** like in **chapter 4.8.**

Note 1: CAUTION: Please don`t manipulate other people. You can operate this exercise also for others, but not without their own wish.

Note 2: The clairvoyant sees how the screens are cleaned and the effects on to the future.

4.4.3.14 Alternative n): Cleaning of the consciousness

Steps	Cleaning
ENT	**Entry** like in example **ENT1 + ENT2**
FOC	**Focusing** like in example **FOC1 (F1-F5)**
CLE	**Cleaning steps:**
C1	„I take a divinely pure screen to my hand."
C2	„I place this divinely pure screen in front of every **screen and** every **mirror of my consciousness** now."
C3	„This screen shall lead all screens and mirrors to divine purity and establish the norm of the Creator within me."
SEC	**Transmission:** like in **chapter 4.7.1.**
EXI	**Exit:** like in **chapter 4.8.**

Note 1: CAUTION: Please don`t manipulate other people. You can operate this exercise also for others, but not without their own wish.

Note 2: The clairvoyant sees how the screens are cleaned and the effects on to the future.

4.5 The Diagnosis Phase (DIA)

4.5.1 <u>Notes</u>

4.5.1.1 We can **diagnose mentally** in many different ways:

- **By** concentration on fingers (= feeling)
- **By** the 3rd eye and analysis of time
- **By** the 3rd eye and direct analysis of the organs, cells, cell nucleuses, chakras etc.
- **By** the 3rd eye and analysis of colors
- **By** automatic, permanent diagnostics by the consciousness e.g. during the night

4.5.1.2 It is <u>not</u> recommended to execute a diagnosis <u>without</u> a previous cleaning.
For many the information of a damage would be hard to differ from some <u>short-term</u> negative information there.

4.5.1.3 Mental diagnosis has different standards of execution. It is possible for most people to notice the vibration of a finger as an indicator, but the 3rd eye is not given to everybody. In addition, the one who sees clairvoyantly not only needs a clear visibility, but also experience in the validity of the seen images.

4.5.2 The Overview of the Alternatives of the Diagnosis (DIA1)

Alternatives	Methods of mental diagnosis
a)	Concentration on certain body segments by finger
b)	Concentration by 2 forefingers and evaluation of the parallelepiped
c)	Perception of the white light at night
d)	Perception of colors
e)	Mental diagnosis by clairvoyance in the organ

Note 1: Alternative c) is an **automatically permanent diagnosis** during the sleep by subconscious **which also functions directly corrective. A very advantageous method!**

Since we feel or see nothing in doing so, **alternative c)** is handled **in chapter 4.6.5. There it is about restoration.**

4.5.3 The partial Steps of the Diagnosis (DIA2) in 5 Alternatives

4.5.3.1 Alternative a): Concentration on certain body segments by finger

Steps	Diagnosis
ENT	**Entry** like in example **ENT1 + ENT2**
FOC	**Focusing** like in example **FOC1 (F1-F5)**
CLE	**Cleaning** like in **chapter 4.4.3.**
DIA	**Diagnosis steps:**
D1	„I am partitioning the body into 10 segments."
D2	„The segment of the soles of the foot corresponds to my little finger on the left."
•	
D4	„The segment „lower part of the pelvis" corresponds to my middle finger."
•	
D11	„The segment „top of the head" corresponds to my right little finger."
D12	„I concentrate on the 2 thumbs now, then on the 2 big toes. Now I listen to myself."
D13	„If a finger answers, I concentrate on the assigned body segment."
SEC	**Transmission:** like in **chapter 4.7.1.**
EXI	**Exit:** like in **chapter 4.8.**

Note 1: This exercise makes it possible to feel a change in the body. **The feeling alone suffices for that.** We don't need clairvoyance here.

Note 2: The perception usually is already the solution of the problem. 6) If any finger answers during our concentration, then we feel a prickling or e.g. warmth. Then we draw attention to the corresponding segment of the body.

Note 3: The segments were defined by Grigori Grabovoi and are well described graphically at Svetlana Smirnova. 12) + 23)

Note 4: The segments which are assigned to a finger here can be further detailed e.g. to a cell or even more detailed to a micro element.

Note 5: A good measure for prevention.

Note 6: The clairvoyant sees how geometries remodel at the respective finger and knows that the right thing happens. He/She also can see the answering finger flashing up.

Note 7: Please take the steps **D3** und **D5-D10** in accordance with **Note 3**.

native b): Concentration on 2 forefingers + evaluation of
ıiped

Steps	Diagnosis
ENT	**Entry** like in example **ENT1 + ENT2**
FOC	**Focusing** like in example **FOC1 (F1-F5)**
CLE	**Cleaning** like in **chapter 4.4.3.**
DIA	**Diagnosis steps:**
D1	„I concentrate on both forefingers."
D2	„I think of my health problem in the organ „Y"."
D3	„I imagine at the same time how a ray comes from each forefinger and both rays meet in front of the thyroid gland in a ball."
D4	„I see the geometry in the ball."
D5	„Restoration of the parallelepiped according to the norm of the Creator: 2 cm wide, 3 cm high, 4 cm deep."
SEC	**Transmission:** like in **chapter 4.7.1.**
EXI	**Exit:** like in **chapter 4.8.**

Note 1: You will find the proper graphic at Hugin Munin. [20]

Note 2: Since the perception often causes a solution already, it is easy to apply for the norm in **D5.**

Note 3: The non-clairvoyant can also apply for the norm.

The non-clairvoyant should nevertheless say the sentence in step **D4,** because voicing brings the geometry on the plan.

Note 4: The clairvoyant sees the parallelepiped in the ball.

The structure represents the time for man. We see the course of the future health.

Note 5: A method very easy to handle for the correction. If we manage the parallelepiped to reach its standard measures, then the connected organ system will also be lead to the norm.

Note 6: The extent of the deformation of the geometry leads to the size of the problems.

Note 7: 10 p.m. – 10.05 p.m. is the best time (see chapter 9 „Unified System of Knowledge"). [6]

4.5.3.3 Alternative c): Diagnostics by perception of the white light at night

Steps	Diagnosis
ENT	**Entry** like in example **ENT1 + ENT2**
FOC	**Focusing** like in example **FOC1 (F1-F5)**
CLE	**Cleaning** like in **chapter 4.4.3.**
DIA	**Diagnosis steps *)**
SEC	**Transmission:** like in **chapter 4.7.1.**
EXI	**Exit:** like in **chapter 4.8.**

Note 1: This diagnosis runs in the context of restoration, since the diagnosis cannot be done consciously.

Note 2: *) See chapter 4.6.5.1.

4.5.3.4 Alternative c): Diagnosis by perception of colors

Steps	Diagnosis
ENT	**Entry** like in example **ENT1 + ENT2**
FOC	**Focusing** like in example **FOC1 (F1-F5)**
CLE	**Cleaning** like in **chapter 4.4.3.**
DIA	**Diagnosis steps**
SEC	**Transmission:** like in **chapter 4.7.1.**
EXI	**Exit:** like in **chapter 4.8.**

Note 1: Colors are suitable for diagnosis very well. They are a reliable tool for the self-knowledge of man. But most individuals can`t see colors with the 3rd eye.

Note 2: What often appears to be difficult here in the diagnosis, then becomes very easy at the control by colors later. **Beause:** We don`t have to see the colors for that.

Thus: The topic „color" **is covered** at the controls **in chapter 4.6.5.**

4.5.3.5 Alternative e): Mental diagnosis by clairvoyance directly to the organ

Steps	Diagnosis
ENT	**Entry** like in example **ENT1 + ENT2**
FOC	**Focusing** like in example **FOC1 (F1-F5)**
CLE	**Cleaning** like in **chapter 4.4.3.**
DIA	**Diagnosis steps:**
D1	„Please show all cells of the hypophysis."
D2	„Please show all cells of the area in the back of the head."
D3	„Please show all cells of the right and left brain hemisphere."
D4	„Please show all cells of the thyroid gland."
D5	„Please show all cells of the central nervous system and the spinal column."
D6	„Please show all cells of the liver."
D7	„Please show all cells of the peripheral nervous system in the head."
D8	Etc.
SEC	**Transmission:** like in **chapter 4.7.1.**
EXI	**Exit:** like in **chapter 4.8.**

Note 1: This mental diagnosis applies only to the practiced persons.

Note 2: The clairvoyant sees e.g. different levels of brightness (from black to very bright), or certain damaged spots, or the cells or the partial areas in a cell down to the DNA-level etc.

Note 3: The clairvoyant can see e.g., if the muscle tissue (after an operatively removed tumor in the bladder) which encloses the bladder, is already attacked at the fine material levels.

Note 4: The clairvoyant should never „go into" a heavy dark event and just watch from the side and from the outside.

Note 5: A really gifted clairvoyant makes interventions and changes so to speak „live". The cooperation with a clairvoyant is not only relieving, but also increases the effectiveness.

4.6 The Restoration Phase (RES)

4.6.1 <u>Notes</u>

•The alternatives are divided in 4 groups: **part I, part II, part III, part IV.**

• You will find the numbers for the restoration of parts of the body, e.g. a muscle, a tooth, the skin etc. in „**Restoration of the Matter by Concentration on Numbers, Volumes I+II".** 14)

• But if there is an **illness,** e.g. a process, we will find the numbers in the book „**Restoration of the human Organism by Concentration on Numbers".** 15)

• The **steps** of this restoration phase also follow the sample worked out before in the chapters „Cleaning" and „Diagnosis".

• The number of alternatives is very extensive. Thank God. Since the body is a holistic system, usually there are many ways of restoration at the mental level for the same problem. **Nevertheless some methods are better than others for the solution of a problem as experience shows.**

• Of course the approaches from „**System of the Education"** 17) can also be used in this phase of restoration. With education system is meant „forming". Here also counts the question: „What is this method particularly well suitable for?"

• Besides, all methods of **resurrection** can be used in the phase of restoration, **e.g. the resurrection of a destroyed cell.**

• In addition, **the placing of new acting principles** is also recommended here.

Question: Why should we do that?

Answer: For example to change our character which also usually is the cause of our illness.

• The exercises from the book „**Concentration Exercises**" can be included here.

• The various **overviews in** the now following **chapter 4.6.2** serve the **easy discovery** (of a matching method or the description of a method).

CAUTION: Who has skipped the chapters of pre-phase, entry phase, focusing, cleaning and diagnosis doesn`t do any favor to himself. Above all, he does not have to be surprised if the wanted results <u>don`t</u> come up.

4.6.2 Overviews of the Alternatives of Restoration (RES)

4.6.2.1 Overview of the Alternatives in Chapter 4.6.3, 4.6.4, 4.6.5 and 4.6.6.

Part I: Alternatives in Chapter 4.6.3

Alternative		Methods of the restoration (shortcut: RES)
a)	**Example of combination**	RES of matter, e.g. hearing organ, and at an illness process, e.g. otitis, by sphere + number sequence
b)	" "	RES, when e.g. sleep disorder, by number and by resurrection (e.g. of the controls)
c)	" "	RES e.g. by doubleganger, e.g. at organ loss
d1)	**Psyche / character / properties**	Resurrection e.g. of consciousness / Christ-consciousness within us
d2)	" "	Resurrection of cosmic consciousness in man ($\rightarrow$ see **picture 1**)
e)	" "	RES of the standard, e.g. in the issue ‚aggression‘ , by number sequence
f)	" "	Dissolving of simple negative events (slight shock, missteps, etc.)
g)	" "	Using of a sphere with a special order by a new principle, e.g. opening for the feeling of love (new property)
h)	" "	Change of character: by „System of Education“
i)	**Psyche / character / properties**	**To acquire new skills:**
i1)	" "	- To refer by yourself to an **example** of „Practice of the Control“: acquisition of clairvoyance
i2)	" "	- New view of life by changing the time configuration (in case of a serious illness such as cancer and life dissatisfaction or e.g. burnout)

i3)	" "	- Restoration of the psyche by concentration on a picture ($\rightarrow$ see picture 2)
j)	**Various illnesses**	RES of organs existing **in pairs** (e.g. kidneys) + vitalization
k1)	" "	- Rejuvenation by numbers and photo
k2)	" "	- Rejuvenation by numbers with plant / crystal
l1)	" "	Damage of **spinal column** (curvature) etc.
l2)	" "	RES of the spinal disc by 4 spheres
l3)	" "	Whole RES of the spinal column by light spheres next to the body
m)	" "	Resurrection, e.g.in case of tinnitus, endocrine problems
n)	" "	Normalization by **double cone** and the number „8" (illness, pain, blood pressure…)
o1)	" "	RES of the digestive system by cylinder-sheet-ball
o2)	" "	To put the Christ-consciousness over an organ
o3)	" "	To put Christ-consciousness from foot to head
p1)	" "	RES of vision (I)
p2)	" "	" " (II)
p3)	" "	" " (III)
p4)	" "	" " (IV) in serious cases
q)	**Various diseases + cancer**	RES **of biopolar signals** (cancer, Parkinson`s)
r)	**Cancer**	To delete ill structures and **central cells**
s)	" "	The removal of cancer cells by sky perspective
t)	" "	RES by reference to the book „Practice of the Control" volume 3 (for cancer)
u)	" "	The change of information about an ill organ in the creative area
v)	" "	To create a **rescuer cell** with a number sequence (Grigori Grabovoi$\rightarrow$ activated structure of coordinates)

w)	" "	Cube-cone-cube and standard cell of the Creator for blood, lymph...
x)	" "	**The control of situations** which have gone out of control (drugs, ...), situations without progress etc.
y)	" "	RES of man from the most serious illness by concentration on a picture ($\rightarrow$ see **picture 3**)

Note 1: RES stands for restoration.

Part II: Alternatives (for the Control of Events) in Chapter 4.6.4

Alternative	Aim	Methods of restoration (RES)
aa)	To produce events	To aim events by concentration on number „3"
ab)	„ „	To control with the help of number „8"
ac)	„ „	To control with the help of sounds waves
ad)	„ „	RES of events / state by concentration exercises for 31 days
ae)	„ „	Solution/ harmonization of a situation by a curved light column
af)	„ „	To realize an event by concentration on a picture ($\rightarrow$ see **picture 4**).

Note 1: These exercises are oriented to generally produce an event or an aim achievement, not only in the health area.

Note 2: The variety makes it easy for us to be reminded of our task of the permanent control by normal daily events again and again.

Part III: Alternatives (special Solutions) in Chapter 4.6.5

Alternative	Aim	Methods of restoration (RES)
ba)	Solution for a special purpose	Perception of the white light at night
bb)	„ „	Allround-method with 2 light columns , e.g. to remove disharmonies or to acquire an ability
bc)	„ „	To „tap" knowledge
bd)	„ „	To get an organ to the norm by **rainbow**-concentration
be)	„ „	Fast searching of the resort by ball on head and in front of the root of the nose
bf)	„ „	To make my reality eternal
bg)	„ „	Special dealing with numbers for the psychological standardization
bh)	„ „	To achieve the aim by self-defined number sequences

Part IV: Alternatives of the <u>complex</u> Restoration in Chapter 4.6.6

Alternative	Aim	Complex restoration
ca)	To build up an ability	→ with 18 different methods
cb)	The complexity in an apparently simple issue	At the examples: - toothache - marriage problems
cc)	An own area of space/time	Make and use of a space/time area for the acquisition of an ability
cd)	**Correction of massive problems from mistakes**	By absolution and repentance….
ce)	Perfect embodiment of the Creator's norm	„To be in paradise" by concentration on a picture (→ see **picture 5**)

4.6.2.2 Overview of the Alternatives of Restoration with Key Points for Part I, II, III and IV

A - Z		In part:
A	acoustic organ	I a)
	aggression	I e)
	Akasha	III bc)
	aging	I k1) + k2)
B	ball on head and in front of the root of the nose	III be)
	bipolar signals	I q)
	brain	Ij) + I p3)
	blood	I w)
	blood pressure	I n)
	burnout / CFS	I i2)
C	change of character	I h) + chapter 4.6.6.4.
	creative area	I t)
	Christ consciousness	I o2) + I o3) + I d1)
	chest	I w)
	cell of God	→ cleaning
	cell with living matter	I r)
	cylinder-sheet-ball	I o1)
	clairvoyance	I i1) + IV ca)
	cleaning	See chapter 4.4.
	control of events	II aa) – af)
	controls of the body	I b)
	color	III bb)

	complex issues	IV ca) – IV ce)
	cancer	I i2) + I q) + I r) + I s) + I t) + I u) + I v) + I y)
	cube-cone-cube	I w)
	color (rainbow)	III bd)
	color white	III ba)
	coccyxs	I q)
D	dissolving information massiveness	I f)
	diagnostic capability	I i1)
	disharmony by color	III bb)
	doubleganger	I c)
	double cone	I n)
	dying	→ not dying
	drugs	I x)
	digestion	I o1)
E	eyes	I p1) – p4) + III bg)
	endocrine system (chest)	I w)
	events	II aa) - II af)
	eight (= number 8)	I n) + II ab)
F	first cell	I r)
	finger-concentration 1	→ diagnosis
	finger-concentration 2 / paired organs	I j)
	fast processes	III ba)
G	Grigori Grabovoi (to understand his teaching)	IV ca)
	greed	I i3)

H	harmonization	IV ce)
	hearing organ	I a)
	humility	III bh)
I / J	information massiveness	I f) + I r) + I u) + IV cd)
	information structure	I r)
	intuition	IV cc)
K	karma	IV cd)
	knowledge	III bc)
L	light column	III bb)
	lighting current	III bb) + cleaning
	love	I g)
	life dissatisfaction	I i2)
	liver	I y)
	lymph	I w)
	leader cell in case of cancer	I r) + I u)
	lost the control (over a situation)	I x)
M	massive problems	IV cd)
	marriage problems	IV cb)
N	not-dying	III bg)
	number „3"	II aa)
	number „8"	I n) + II ab)
	number sequence	I a) + I b) + I e) + I p1) + I v) + III bg) + III bh) + IV cc)
O	ozone	→ cleaning
	organ loss	I c)

	organ restoration	I o2)
	otitis	I a)
P	paired organs	I j)
	parallelepiped	→ diagnosis
	Parkinson`s	I q)
	principle (new) – to put	I g)
	put an ability	I i1 + III bb) + III bf) + IV ca) + IV cc)
	problems, massive	IV cd)
	psyche	I i3) + III bb) + III bf) + III bg) + IV ce)
	pain	I n)
	pictures	I d2) + I i3) + I y) + II af) + IV ce)
	property (→ see ‚put an ability‘)	I c)
Q		
R	rejuvenation	I k1) + k2)
	reality: to make it eternal	III bf)
	rainbow	III bd)
	rescuer cell	I v) + i p2)
	refer to „Practice of the control“	I i1) + I t)
	raising consciousness	I d)
	raising of Christ consciousness	I d1)
	raising of cosmic consciousness	I d2)
	raising / endocrine system (chest)	I m)
	raising vision	I p3)

	raising / controls	I b)
	raising / tinnitus	I m)
	raising cells / connections / areas in the brain and spinal cord	I p3)
S	standard cell of God	I v)
	sound waves	II ac)
	sleep disorder	I b)
	source of the negative	I q)
	system of education	I h)
	space/ time area	IV cc)
	searching of resort	III be)
	shock (to dissolve))	I f)
	soul (cleaning)	→ cleaning
	spinal cord	I p3)
	situation out of control	I x)
	spine – spinal disc	I l2)
	spine - curvature	I l1)
	spine – complete spine	I l3)
T	tinnitus	I m)
	thyroid gland	II ac)
	teeth	IV cb)
	time configuration	I i2)
	three (= number 3)	II aa)
U	urogenital area	I j)
V	vertebra	I q)
	vision	I p1) – p4) + III bg)
W	white light	III ba)
X , Y, Z		

4.6.3. The partial Steps of the Restoration (Part I), represented in 33 Alternatives (RES2)

4.6.3.1. Alternative a): Restoration of matter, e.g. (hearing and equilibrium organ) and of a disease (e.g. otitis)

Steps	Restoration
ENT	**Entry** like in example **ENT1 + ENT2**
FOC	**Focusing** like in example **FOC1 (F1-F5)**
CLE	**Cleaning** like in **chapter 4.4.3.**
DIA	**Diagnosis steps** like in **chapter 4.5.3.**
RES-I	**Main steps:**
R1	„Restoration of all cells of the hearing and equilibrium organ to the norm of the Creator: * I place the number sequence 248 712 on the left side of the person and on the right 318 222. * Christ, please give light to this **number sequence**, so that its shadow can cause the best effect on person ‚XY‘. * The materializing takes place in front of the background of the soul of the Creator."
R2	„Light sphere, please, in front of the right forefinger."
R3	„I place into the light sphere the impulses: - Golden light, love, harmony, luck, joy of the eternal further development and - the **number sequence** 55184321."
R4	„Please shrink the light sphere to 1 point."
R5	„Transfer to the pituitary." + **Impulse**
SEC	**Transmission:** like in **chapter 4.7.1.**
EXI	**Exit:** like in **chapter 4.8.**

Note 1: You will find the numbers for **R1** in „**Restoration of the matter…**"[14)]

Note 2: The number in **R3** relates to a **process** of "**otitis**" and not on a matter like in **R1**. Therefore this number is in the book "**Restoration of the human Organism…**"[15)]

Note 3: Please also compare the **restoration by raising** (e.g. in case of tinitus) → see chapter 4.6.3.16.

Note 4: We mentally give the impulse in **R5** over the forefinger right and respectively an impulse in **R3** in each term.

Note 5: The mental imagination for placing the numbers in **R3** could also be done like in the book "Concentration Exercises"[16)].

4.6.3.2. Alternative b): Restoration by number (e.g.in case of sleep disorder) + raising (e.g. of the controls)

Steps	Restoration
ENT	**Entry** like in example **ENT1 + ENT2**
FOC	**Focusing** like in example **FOC1 (F1-F5)**
CLE	**Cleaning** like in **chapter 4.4.3.**
DIA	**Diagnosis steps** like in **chapter 4.5.3.**
RES-I	**Main steps:**
R1	„Light sphere please in front of the right forefnger."
R2	„I give the folowing impulses into the light sphere: - golden light - love - harmony - luck - joy of the eternal further development."
R3	„I also place the **number sequence** 514248538 into the sphere."
R4	„Shrinking of the light sphere to pea size and transfer it by light connection to the small right finger ."
R5	„I transmit to the infinity for an infinite further development." +
R6	**„Impulse."** **Note:** To give an impulse and to send the sphere to an infinitely far away point.
R7	„**Raising** of all connections and controls within person XY to the norm of the Creator. **Raising** of all functions within XY which are connected with sleep disorders. **Raising** of all these functions and eternal life of these functions within XY."
SEC	**Transmission:** like in **chapter 4.7.1.**
EXI	**Exit:** like in **chapter 4.8.**

Note 1: At **R6** the imagination helps that the sphere disappears in a point on a railroad in the distance.

Note 2: The word **"raising"** has to be spoken in a certain way, namely in a cantation manner. And then absolutely always 3-fold.

Note 3: The clairvoyant sees at the raising here e.g.how a sphere becomes transparent, remodels into a transparent cubus and manifests with that and becomes very bright.

4.6.3.3. Alternative c): Restoration by doubleganger e.g. in case of organ loss of the gall

Steps	Restoration
ENT	**Entry** like in example **ENT1 + ENT2**
FOC	**Focusing** like in example **FOC1 (F1-F5)**
CLE	**Cleaning** like in **chapter 4.4.3.**
DIA	**Diagnosis steps** like in **chapter 4.5.3.**
RES-I	**Main steps:**
R1	„I transfer the time of person XY to 10 p.m. of Moscow time.“ + impulse
R2	„And now I give a double impulse on the right forefinger.”
R3	„Light sphere, please, from the ultra-distant area in front of the right forefinger.”
R4	„I place into the light sphere the impulses: Golden light, love, harmony, luck and joy of the eternal further development.“
R5	„**Doubleganger** in accordance with prototype of person XY, please.“
R6	„Direct light connection between the gall in the prototype and the sphere in front of the right forefinger.“
R7	„Load all the information and its connections from the prototype into the sphere .“
R8	„A **copy of the sphere**, please and shrinking to pea size. Transfer of the copy to the place of the gall.“ + impulse
R9	„Shrink the **original sphere** to a point and transfer into the pituitary.“
R10	„The pituitary takes the control over the new sphere of the gall. Light arrow with white light from the pituitary to the new sphere of the gall.“
R11	„**Convert** this **sphere** to the new first cell of the gall.“
R12	„Restoration of all cells of the gall to the norm of the Creator and reproduction of the first cell according to the Fibonacci-number sequence“ + **Impulse**
SEC	**Transmission:** like in **chapter 4.7.1.**
EXI	**Exit:** like in **chapter 4.8.**

Note 1: This example was built up in that way that everybody is able to recognize what is possible.

Note 2: If this example were built up directly with a cell from the ultra-distant area, then some steps would be different of course.

Note 3: It goes without saying that such a process requires a support again and again.

Note 4: The clairvoyant sees e.g. a transparent cube as a sign of materialization.

4.6.3.4. Alternative d1): Raising e.g. of the Christ Consciousness + the health within us

Steps	Restoration
ENT	**Entry** like in example **ENT1 + ENT2**
FOC	**Focusing** like in example **FOC1 (F1-F5)**
CLE	**Cleaning** like in **chapter 4.4.3.**
DIA	**Diagnosis Steps** like in **chapter 4.5.3.**
RES-I	**Main Steps:**
R1	„**Raising** of the Christ Consciousness within person XY."
R2	„**Raising** of the Christ Consciousness within all cells and Controls of XY."
R3	„**Raising** of the Christ Consciousness within all cells and Controls of XY and eternal life of the Christ Consciousness and these functions in XY. "
R4	„Cleaning and restoration of all my displays with the Christ Consciousness to the norm of the Creator."
SEC	**Transmission:** like in **chapter 4.7.1.**
EXI	**Exit:** like in **chapter 4.8.**

Note 1: A very easy exercise, but very efficient.

Note 2: Since it is the task of man that we develop in the direction of Christ more and more, this alternative is a very important opportunity for the realization.

Note 3: In addition, this exercise cleans up within us and with that it is **one of the most important methods for the elimination of illnesses.**

Note 4: Experience shows that the 3-fold repetition of the word **"raising"** is absolutely necessary in an incantation manner.

Note 5: The clairvoyant sees e.g. a variety of truthful Christ symbols and the joy of the cells. The clearing up of past burdens we can see e.g. in a picture of the toes on the left which then are represented very brightly.

Note 6: The dealing with the issue "raising" should be part of the daily repertoire.

Because: Every restoration leads to a clearing up also at another place in universe.

Note 7: A negative information massiveness usually can`t be removed by raising. See to that 4.6.3.16. Note 5.

4.6.3.5. Alternative d2): Raising of the Cosmic Consciousness within man by concentration on a picture

Steps	Restoration
ENT	**Entry** like in example **ENT1 + ENT2**
FOC	**Focusing** like in example **FOC1 (F1-F5)**
CLE	**Cleaning** like in **chapter 4.4.3.**
DIA	**Diagnosis Steps** like in **chapter 4.5.3.**
RES-I	**Main Steps:**
R1	„I concentrate on the picture for raising of the Cosmic Consciousness within man."
R2	„Now I let the picture take effect on me and ask for ..." (e.g. extended access to the Cosmic Consciousness)
SEC	**Transmission:** like in **chapter 4.7.1.**
EXI	**Exit:** like in **chapter 4.8.**

Note 1: The title of the picture is **"Raising of the Cosmic Consciousness within man"**.

Note 2: See chapter 4.1.3 e) for picture contemplation.

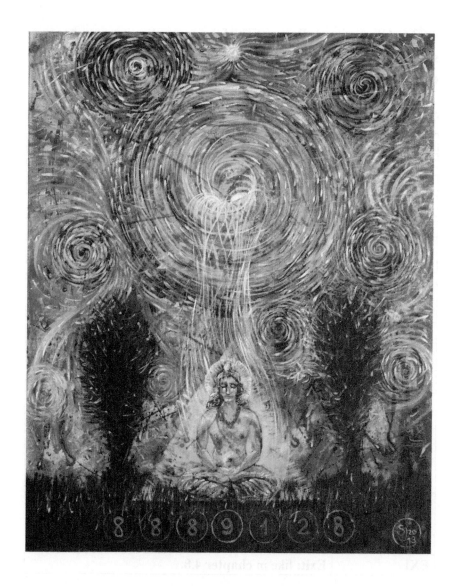

Sergey Jelezky, Öl auf Leinwand,
100x80cm, 2013

4.6.3.6. Alternative e): Restoration of the norm of an issue e.g. "aggression" and restoration of the norm in accordance with the norm of the Creator for all events of the issue "aggression"

Steps	Restoration
EIN	**Entry** like in example **ENT1 + ENT2**
FOK	**Focusing** like in example **FOC1 (F1-F5)**
REI	**Cleaning** like in **chapter 4.4.3.**
DIA	**Diagnosis Steps** like in **chapter 4.5.3.**
RES-I	**Main Steps:**
R1	„I load into the sphere on the forfinger **left** the issue ‚aggression'."
R2	(For clairvoyants): „I ask for information concerning the status of the condition of this issue. Christ ‚please, help."
R3	„I place the **number sequence** ‚5,2,8...,'....etc."
R4	„Christ, please, give divine light on this number sequence (within person XY) so that the best effect can be achieved."
R5	„The materializing takes place in front of the background of the soul of the Creator."
R6	„Restoration of the norm of the Creator **for the issue** ‚aggression',, or: „Restoration of the norm of the Creator **for all events** of the issue ‚aggression'."
SEC	**Transmission:** like in **chapter 4.7.1.**
EXI	**Exit:** like in **chapter 4.8.**

Note 1: Who doesn`t see clairvoyantly, just leaves out step **R2.**

Note 2: The experience and observation of clairvoyants show that in each person much more psycho issues are in a sad state than you could think first.

Note 3: The situation becomes considerably better within the person relating to this issue with increasing and repeated retrieving and processing.

Note 4: We cannot dissolve enough issues at all. Please consider that Grigori Grabovoi has recommended again and again to read and work on every terms, at least for once.

Note 5: You will find the number sequences in the "Psycho-Guide" by Grigori Grabovoi. 26) It is worthwile to look there.

4.6.3.7. Alternative f): Dissolving of simple negative events/ simple negative information massiveness, like e.g. smaller shocks, mistakes etc.

Steps	Restoration
ENT	**Entry** like in example **ENT1 + ENT2**
FOC	**Focusing** like in example **FOC1 (F1-F5)**
CLE	**Cleaning** like in **chapter 4.4.3.**
DIA	**Diagnosis Steps** like in **chapter 4.5.3.**
RES-I	**Main Steps:**
R1	„I load into the sphere in front of the forefinger **left** my relation to the mother-in-law Martha Dispute."
R2	„I`m asking you, Martha Dispute, let off so that we can go into the light. I forgive you and you also please forgive me."
R3	„Please, Christ, help that all persons involved can go into the light. I`m asking for the takeover of all negative burdens to the divine level for the transfer into the light."
R4	„I send my love from the heart so that the process may run easier, at first to the Creator and then to all persons involved."
R5	Etc. etc.
SEC	**Transmission:** like in **chapter 4.7.1.**
EXI	**Exit:** like in **chapter 4.8.**

Note 1: Read to this in Grigori Grabovoi supplementarily. 8)

Note 2: It should be clear that the heaviest negative events of the past require more steps and more effort. **See to that e.g. chapter 4.6.6.4.**

Note 3: The problem: **We all are much more involved in certain issues than we might think first!** And many people think they already have dissolved their problems with the one or other method. This is a mistake in most cases.

Note 4: The clairvoyant sees the picture of a situation, matching the issue. And the pictures change with the progress of the issue.

Note 5: Furthermore, it should be clear that every step <u>always</u> gives an effect. **Who doesn`t see anything** could let himself be guided by his feeling (but please without any self-cheating). The work is only done when we have attained a completely neutral relation to the respective event or to the person after the session and when nothing dark shows up clairvoyantly any more.

4.6.3.8. Alternative g): A sphere with a special order e.g. "opening for the feeling of love"

Steps	Restoration
ENT	**Entry** like in example **ENT1 + ENT2**
FOC	**Focusing** like in example **FOC1 (F1-F5)**
CLE	**Cleaning** like in **chapter 4.4.3.**
DIA	**Diagnosis Steps** like in **chapter 4.5.3.**
RES-I	**Main Steps:**
R1	„I concentrate on the forefinger **right**.“
R2	„Light spehre, please, 1 cm of diameter.“
R3	„Input: silvery, white light of the Creator.“
R4	„All inputs in canonical shape.“
R5	„Impulses of love, harmony, luck and the joy of eternal further development.“
R6	„The sphere gets the order: opening for the feeling of love.“
R7	"Effect from now on up to eternity.“
R8	„Golden light of the Creator.“ + **Impulse**
R9	„Transfer of the sphere next to person XY, on the right of his/her head, please.“ + to give an **impulse**
SEC	**Transmission:** like in **chapter 4.7.1.**
EXI	**Exit:** like in **chapter 4.8.**

Note 1: Plese read to this Grigori Grabovoi 32) about the effect of such spheres.

Note 2: With this methods we place a new "principle".

Note 3: To **R2:** imagine the sphere about 1 cm in front of the forefinger right.

Note 4: To **R5, R8** and **R9:** To send impulses by forefinger on the right.

Note 5: The clairvoyant not only sees the light sphere, but also a picture for the content of the placed order. **Caution** is advisable with the choice of the order because what we want for others could already fulfill the fact of manipulation of other persons. **But with love we can`t do anything wrong.**

Note 6: The placing of such spheres often brings amazing effects.

Note 7: A sphere in front of us changes the existing, the sphere next to us gives "new things".

4.6.3.9. Alternative h): Change of character by System of Education

Steps	Restoration
ENT	**Entry** like in example **ENT1 + ENT2**
FOC	**Focusing** like in example **FOC1 (F1-F5)**
CLE	**Cleaning** like in **chapter 4.4.3.**
DIA	**Diagnosis Steps** like in **chapter 4.5.3.**
RES-I	**Main-Steps:**
R1	**Note 1:** Look at the work ,Educational System' by Grigori Grabovoi.17) + 22)
	Note 2: The work gives good instructions for changing something and for"openings" of the personal-emotional area.
	Note 3: The method listed there shows how we can lead **ourselves or others** to positive, constructive positions by dialogue and how we can develop the personality. The observed changes are amazing in many cases.
	Note 4: An unusual feature is that this method works **independently** of the **age** of a person.

	Note 5: In addition, we can start at any time chosen, also before birth or in the future. I.e. we are able to change something even years before birth to cause a change of the world view of person XY. On the other hand we can already today form the behavior of the future of person XY in
	Note 6: Manipulation is <u>not</u> done here. The necessary texts are provided by Grigori Grabovoi.
	Note 7: Since serious illnesses are associated with personal-emotional problems, we can **show the optimal way** with this approach **to the soul.**
	Note 8: It is clear that a young person or an unborn one is easier to be lead on the right way than an older person.
SEC	**Transmission:** like in **chapter 4.7.1.**
EXI	**Exit:** like in **chapter 4.8.**

4.6.3.10. Alternative i1): Acquisition of a new ability (here e.g. clairvoyance) by referring yourself on an example of "Practice of the Control"

Steps	Restoration
ENT	**Entry** like in example **ENT1 + ENT2**
FOC	**Focusing** like in example **FOC1 (F1-F5)**
CLE	**Cleaning** like in **chapter 4.4.3.**
DIA	**Diagnosis Steps** like in **chapter 4.5.3.**
RES-I	**Main Steps:**
R1	„Please hear me, Christ."
R2	„I´m asking for help so that I am able to better help others."
R3	„I am asking for the gift of clairvoyance, to be able to exactly **determine** the outward appearance and the **character of a person without** having some preliminary **information** about this person."
R4	„In addition, I am asking to be able to exactly **diagnose** mentally from any chosen **distance.**"
R5	„I´m asking to be able to develop these abilities analogous to the document that is described on the pages… in the work ‚Praxis der Steuerung, Weg der Rettung, volume 2' by Grigori Grabovoi in the German translation in the 1st edition of October 2011."
R6	„Grigori Grabovoi, please hear me and support this process."
SEC	**Transmission:** like in **chapter 4.7.1.**
EXI	**Exit:** like in **chapter 4.8.**

Note 1: The work „Praxis der Steuerung" (Practice of the Control) volume 2 offers a lot of examples of <u>special</u> abilities which we could acquire.

Note 2: The work "Practice of the Control" make it able for us to refer to it. Therefore they are part of the "medicine chest".

Note 3: Please also read what is written in Hugin Munin to that. [21]

Note 4: To the clairvoyant could appear e.g. a pigeon (Holy Ghost) or also a red carpet or the like which introduces the process. **If the called ones appear, then the support will be there, too, in case... → see prerequisites.**

Note 5: In **R5** we, of course, have to cite the selected side then.

4.6.3.11. Alternative i2): To change time configuration in case of serious illness (e.g. cancer + life dissatisfaction or by an initiation of it (e.g. burnout))

Steps	Restoration
ENT	**Entry** like in example **ENT1 + ENT2**
FOC	**Focusing** like in example **FOC1 (F1-F5)**
CLE	**Cleaning** like in **chapter 4.4.3.**
DIA	**Diagnosis Steps** like in **chapter 4.5.3.**
RES-I	**Main Steps:**
R1	„I concentrate on the little finger on the right hand from 10 p.m. to 11 p.m."
R2	„I go into a room where everything is harmonious."
R3	"There is no time in this room."
R4	„I feel the whole palette of the harmony of sounds, colors and geometries."
R5	„This is my upcoming world."
R6	„**I hereby decide** to keep the attention on this finger for 3 days."
SEC	**Transmission:** like in **chapter 4.7.1.**
EXI	**Exit:** like in **chapter 4.8.**

Note 1: The time corresponds to <u>German</u> time. We can transfer our time to every other point in time at 10 p.m., analogous to **R1** in **4.6.3.3.**

Note 2: If we take the <u>time out</u> of negatively running processes, then the process stops. This happens with **R3**. The time of execution (i.e. of the process) has nothing to do with the time configuration.

Note 3: An alternative to this is to change the <u>time configuration</u>.

Note 4: The change of time configuration can happen in different ways. E.g. like shown in this example here in a special, harmonizing room.

Note 5: We have to **decide** that our attention will be concentrated on this finger during the 3 days.

Note 6: The clairvoyant sees e.g. a large number of harmonious geometries full of colors. Shamballah can be seen here among others. And the little finger catches fire.

Note 7: Color exercises offer further alternatives of the change of time configuration.

4.6.3.12. Alternative i3): Restoration of the <u>psyche</u> by concentration on a picture

Steps	Restoration
ENT	**Entry** like in example **ENT1 + ENT2**
FOC	**Focusing** like in example **FOC1 (F1-F5)**
CLE	**Cleaning** like in **chapter 4.4.3.**
DIA	**Diagnosis Steps** like in **chapter 4.5.3.**
RES-I	**Main Steps:**
R1	„I concentrate on the picture for the restoration of the psyche."
R2	„I now let the picture take effect on my soul and I ask for..."(e.g. dissolving of my greed)
SEC	**Transmission: like in chapter 4.7.1.**
EXI	**Exit: like in chapter 4.8.**

Note 1: The **title** of the picture is „**Restoration of the Psyche**".

Note 2: See chapter 4.1.3 e) for picture contemplation.

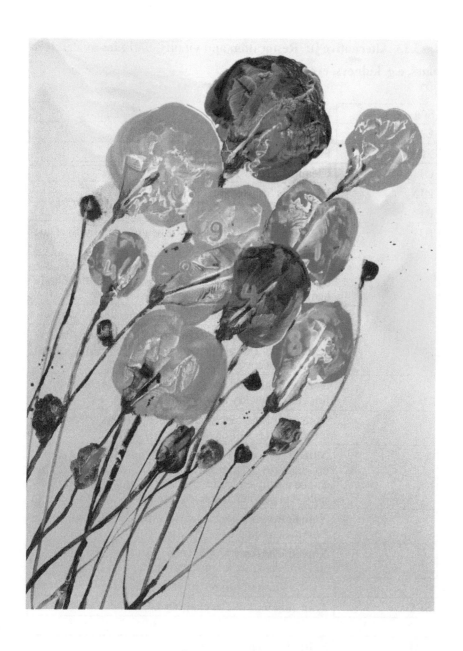

Sergey Jelezky, Öl auf Leinwand, 100x80cm, 2013

4.6.3.13. Alternative j): Restoration and vitality of organs avalaible in pairs, e.g. kidneys, eyes...

Steps	Restoration
ENT	**Entry** like in example **ENT1 + ENT2**
FOC	**Focusing** like in example **FOC1 (F1-F5)**
CLE	**Cleaning** like in **chapter 4.4.3.**
DIA	**Diagnosis Steps** like in **chapter 4.5.3.**
RES-I	**Main Steps:**
R1	**Note 1:** The exercise is documented well by Svetlana Smirnova. 12)
	Note 2: This exercise regenerates and rejuvenates the organs available in pairs. This is also valid for the 2 brain hemispheres.
	Note 3:. In addition, new cells are generated.
	Note 4: Since the function of brain cells is also activated, a further field of application opens: **Refreshing** of our power in case we e.g. are "sagging".
	Note 5: This exercise is based on that we adress the fingers as quickly as possible.
	Note 6: It is not necessary to see the fingers, the mental imagination is sufficient.
	Note 7: The clairvoyant sees e.g. how the order comes up, respectively a picture that indicates the order. This can be a simple picture, e.g. a lot of rods arranged vertically + in parallel next to each other.
	Note 8: An important exercise, especially because of the 2 brain hemispheres.
	Note 9: The daily prophylaxis takes less than 5 minutes and will save us a lot inconvenience.
	Vorstellung reicht vollkommen aus.
SEC	**Transmission:** like in **chapter 4.7.1.**
EXI	**Exit:** like in **chapter 4.8.**

4.6.3.14. Alternative k1): Rejuventaion by numbers and photo Alternative k2): Rejuventaion with plant and crystal

Steps	Restoration
ENT	**Entry** like in example **ENT1 + ENT2**
FOC	**Focusing** like in example **FOC1 (F1-F5)**
CLE	**Cleaning** like in **chapter 4.4.3.**
DIA	**Diagnosis Steps** like in **chapter 4.5.3.**
RES-I	**Main Steps:**
R1	**Note 1:** This exercise is decribed well by Svetlana Smirnova. 1)
	Note 2: Aging is not a natural process. Aging is an illness that is based on wrong will, wrong thinking, wrong feeling and wrong acting and can be reversed..
	Note 3: At this type of exercise, in each case <u>both</u> number sequences should be used.
	Note 4: The variety of different approaches makes it easier for us to be able to practice during the day again and again, because the different occasions run on the road more frequently. There are plants almost everywhere.
	Note 5: The observation shows that people also get to an "internal" rejuvenation in case of visible (to the outside) successes.
	Note 6: The clairvoyant sees e.g. a face without wrinkles as forecast. A statement about the running process could also occur, e.g. a beard and head hair which shorten. Heaven also proves humor in the messages.
	Note 7: In addition, the rejuvenation is also up to a desired age, <u>without</u> thereby setting a mental step backwards.
	Note 8: The exercise fits well to the previous one and lives especially from repetition. The joy of a visible rejuvenation is usually huge.
	Note 9: <u>Again:</u> Aging ist <u>not</u> a natural process, but artificially provoked by us, as well as Alzheimer`s disease is an acquired feeble-mindedness.
SEC	**Transmission:** like in **chapter 4.7.1.**
EXI	**Exit:** like in **chapter 4.8.**

4.6.3.15. Alternative l1): Spinal curvature and intervertebral disc abrasion

Alternative l2): Intervertebral disc slippage and displaced vertebrae (technology of the 4 speheres)

Alternative l3): Full restoration of the spinal column by light spheres at foot-, knee- and hip joint

Steps	Restoration
ENT	**Entry** like in example **ENT1 + ENT2**
FOC	**Focusing** like in example **FOC1 (F1-F5)**
CLE	**Cleaning** like in **chapter 4.4.3.**
DIA	**Diagnosis Steps** like in **chapter 4.5.3.**
RES-I	**Main Steps:**
R1	**Note 1:** These exercises of the alternatives l1 + l2 are described by Svetlana Smirnova very well graphically. 1). You will find the graphic for alternative l3) in the workshop „Basics 2".
	Note 2: Since serious spinal column problems are connected to violations of God first of all, every exercise of regeneration is very important and due to the holographic structure of man much more further reaching than we would think at first.
	Note 3: Changes of the spinal column often have serious consequences. This gets clear when we know that e.g. a disturbed cervical vertebra is also able to disturb the metabolism processes.

	Note 4: By spinal column problems mostly the whole organism is affected. Therefore, we cannot
	Note 5: The technology of the 4 spheres is also suitable very well to expel newly captured negative entities out of the central nervous system. Go on 9/10 of light velocity for the "up- and down rolling".
	Note 6: At least the 4 sphere technology should be used daily.
	Note 7: The clairvoyant sees how other body areas which are in connection with a spinal column part improve with this exercises.
SEC	**Transmission:** like in **chapter 4.7.1.**
EXI	**Exit:** like in **chapter 4.8.**

4.6.3.16. Alternative m): Raising, e.g. in case of tinnitus, endocrine problems

Steps	Restoration
ENT	**Entry** like in example **ENT1 + ENT2**
FOC	**Focusing** like in example **FOC1 (F1-F5)**
CLE	**Cleaning** like in **chapter 4.4.3.**
DIA	**Diagnosis Steps** like in **chapter 4.5.3.**
RES-I	**Main Steps:**
R1	„**Raising** of all cells of the hearing organ of the left head for person XY."
R2	„**Raising** of all cells of the hearing organ of the left head as well as all areas in the brain and in the spinal cord which are connected to it and also the connections themselves there."
R3	„**Raising** of all functions, like said before, **within** person XY and eternal life of this functions within XY."
SEC	**Transmission:** like in **chapter 4.7.1.**
EXI	**Exit:** like in **chapter 4.8.**

Note 1: The word „raising" has to be spoken in a certain way, i.e. in an incantation manner and also 3-fold.

Note 2: The problems in the hearing organ mostly have been built up over a long time: correspondingly the regeneration proceeds **slowly.**

Note 3: The clairvoyant sees very **fast** a stabilization of the aura although fluctuations of the tonality in the ear appear furthermore. The noise level itself goes back only slowly.

Note 4: The causes often are errors in form of hate, criticism of others etc.

Note 5: It is appropriately sensible to **use** here **in parallel** the **methods** of number placing from different areas (illness plus matter plus psycho numbers and also dissolving in accordance with chapter 4.6.6.4). Through that an extremely strong approach arises.

Note 6: This example can be transferred to other parts of the body, e.g. to all cells of the endocrine system of the (left) chest.

Note 7: So where is the problem actually, if a negative appearance needs 2 years to have the negative drained away again?

4.6.3.17. Alternative n): Transformation and lead processes and situations to the norm by double cone and the number "8"

Steps	Restoration
ENT	Entry like in example ENT1 + ENT2
FOC	Focusing like in example FOC1 (F1-F5)
CLE	Cleaning like in chapter 4.4.3.
DIA	Diagnosis Steps like in chapter 4.5.3.
RES-I	Main Steps:
R1	Note 1: As processes we can understand also other processes than diseases, e.g. processes of the daily life.
	Note 2: In contrast unemployment is a situation, not a process.
	Note 3: So, no matter if illness, pain, unemployment, relationship problems, the double cone turns them to normality.
	Note 4: In the geometry of the double spiral a basic structure of the universe becomes visible. Many processes in the universe run after the scheme of the double spiral to initiate something in the zero-point (=meeting point of the 2 spirals).
	Note 5: And the combination with the „8" gives us one of the constructive measures again.
	Note 6: This exercise is described very well by Svetlana Smirnova. 12)

	Note 7: The clairvoyant sees e.g. a matching picture to the element which is connected to the problem brought in, e.g. the ring finger (= air element/communication) at the desire for restoration of the hearing organ.
	Note 8: Furthermore, situations can be stabilized with luck balls. 11)
	Note 9: And we can work on situations with the business numbers very differentiatedly. 25)
SEC	**Transmission:** like in **chapter 4.7.1.**
EXI	**Exit:** like in **chapter 4.8.**

4.6.3.18. Alternative o1): Restoration of the digestion system by cylinder-sheet-ball

Steps	Restoration
ENT	**Entry** like in example **ENT1 + ENT2**
FOC	**Focusing** like in example **FOC1 (F1-F5)**
CLE	**Cleaning** like in **chapter 4.4.3.**
DIA	**Diagnosis Steps** like in **chapter 4.5.3.**
RES-I	**Main Steps:**
R1	**Note 1:** This exercise is also described very well by Svetlana Smirnova. 1)
	Note 2: You will find supplementary information with Grigori Grabovoi. 7) + 8)
	Note 3: The **combination of the removal** of negative information **and the contribution** of the good condition is interesting here.
	Note 4: This method should become a permanent institution at today`s eating habits.
	Note 5: But who then thinks to be safe by the application of this method and to be able to eat the indigestible things now is really mistaken. The divine authorities cannot be duped.
	Note 6: The clairvoyant sees how the cylinder expands by the contribution of negative information. The expansion can take astonishing extents.
	Note 7: The process of negative-drain can also drag on longer from the point of view of time.

	Note 8: This geometry may <u>not</u> be used for any organs but for the tube-shaped parts of the body like veins, lymphatics, intestines, gullet, air tube.
SEC	**Transmission:** like in **chapter 4.7.1.**
EXI	**Exit: like in chapter 4.8.**

4.6.3.19. Alternative o2): To put the Christ Consciousness over an organ

Steps	Restoration
ENT	**Entry** like in example **ENT1 + ENT2**
FOC	**Focusing** like in example **FOC1 (F1-F5)**
CLE	**Cleaning** like in **chapter 4.4.3.**
DIA	**Diagnosis Steps** like in **chapter 4.5.3.**
RES-I	**Main Steps:**
R1	„I put an ‚X' of silvery white light over the organ ‚Z'.
R2	„Restoration to the norm of the Creator."
SEC	**Transmission:** like in **chapter 4.7.1.**
EXI	**Exit:** like in **chapter 4.8.**

Note 1: The restoration of an ill organ to the norm is a little bit different than the raising of a lost organ.

Note 2: It is astonishing how fast the brightness usually returns into the organ.

4.6.3.20. Alternative o3): To put Christ Consciousness from head to feet

Steps	Restoration
ENT	**Entry** like in example **ENT1 + ENT2**
FOC	**Focusing** like in example **FOC1 (F1-F5)**
CLE	**Cleaning** like in **chapter 4.4.3.**
DIA	**Diagnosis Steps** like in **chapter 4.5.3.**
RES-I	**Main Steps:**
R1	„I put an ‚X' of silvery white light from the two soles of the foot to the forehead bumps of my front head."
R2	„Restoration to the norm of the Creator."
SEC	**Transmission:** like in **chapter 4.7.1.**
EXI	**Exit:** like in **chapter 4.8.**

Note 1: An elegant and strong method to bring the brigthness back at once at several places.

Note 2: This solution works, since we automatically achieve the effect at every level by the proper way to enter.

Note 3: CAUTION: The general picture can be alright, even if the detail is not alright.

4.6.3.21. Alternative p1): To restore the vision (I) <u>by sphere</u> with number sequences

Steps	Restoration
ENT	**Entry** like in example **ENT1 + ENT2**
FOC	**Focusing** like in example **FOC1 (F1-F5)**
CLE	**Cleaning** like in **chapter 4.4.3.**
DIA	**Diagnosis Steps** like in **chapter 4.5.3.**
RES-I	**Main Steps:**
R1	„Light sphere with silvery white light in front of the right forefinger, please."
R2	„I put the impulses into the light sphere: - Golden light - Love - Harmony - Luck - Joy of the eternal further development."
R3	„I place the number sequence 1891014 into the sphere."
R4	„I now press the sphere mentally together to the size of a tennis ball."
R5	„Transfer in the middle of the head behind the eyes of person YX, please." + **Impulse**
R6	„The silvery white light now streams out of the sphere like a spotlight out of the eyes."
SEC	**Transmission:** like in **chapter 4.7.1.**
EXI	**Exit:** like in **chapter 4.8.**

Note 1: To remove glasses as **R5.**

Note 2: It shows that the vision usually improves only slowly.

Question: What is this due to?

Answer: The vision is often based on serious violations of the divine order of the universe, as well as the area of the hearing organ. In case of eye problems arrogance (e.g. towards God) is one of the most frequent causes among others, but also bad points such as hate and greed. **If you tidy up in the personal-emotional area, astonishing progresses can be realized.**

Note 3: Please take a look at the chapter "Prerequisites" in this book here. There it becomes clear what is going on with the divine order.

Note 4: Otherwise the in alternative m) said to tinnitus is valid.

Note 5: The clairvoyant sees at this exercise here how the spotlight is shining out of the eyes. Possibly Shiva also appears in the lotus position with a mudra in the right hand.

4.6.3.22. Alternative p2): To restore the vision (II) by rescuer cell

Steps	Restoration
ENT	**Entry** like in example **ENT1 + ENT2**
FOC	**Focusing** like in example **FOC1 (F1-F5)**
CLE	**Cleaning** like in **chapter 4.4.3.**
DIA	**Diagnosis Steps** like in **chapter 4.5.3.**
RES-I	**Main Steps:**
R1	**Note 1: Insert** a **rescuer cell** 12) mentally into the eyeball and reproduce the rescuer cell clockwise.
	Note 2: The graphic of the creation of the rescuer cell is directly explanatory at Svetlana Smirnova. 12)
	Note 3: With this way the ill cells are provided with normizing information by the rescuer cells.
	Note 4: The reproduction takes place best with the Fibonacci-number sequence: 1,1,2,3,5,8,13 etc. Just apply for „reproduction with the Fibonacci-number sequence."
	Note 5: The said in Alternative p1) to Note 2 is also valid here.
	Note 6: Who isn't reasonable doesn't need to complain about his suffering. Insight has something to do with eyesight. Please look at the chapter „Prerequisites" in this book here.
	Note 7: The rescuer cell shows us the importance of love as healing strength.

	Note 8: It is interesting that e.g. exactly this geometry of the rescuer cell can appear to the clairvoyant (at the activation of the cell of God). So this geometry is not an earthly invention but a divine gift.
	Note 9: Please also read to this alternative v).
SEC	Transmission: like in chapter 4.7.1.
EXI	Exit: like in chapter 4.8.

4.6.3.23. Alternative p3): To restore the vision (III) by raising

Steps	Restoration
ENT	**Entry** like in example **ENT1 + ENT2**
FOC	**Focusing** like in example **FOC1 (F1-F5)**
CLE	**Cleaning** like in **chapter 4.4.3.**
DIA	**Diagnosis Steps** like in **chapter 4.5.3.**
RES-I	**Main Steps:**
R1	„Raising of all **cells** of the left rear optic **thalamus**.“
	„Raising of all cells of the **connection** from the left rear optic thalamus to the right eye.“
	„Raising of all **cells** of the right **eye**.“
	„Raising of all **areas** of the **brain** and of the **spinal cord** which are connected to the right eye **and these connections** themselves.“
R2	„Raising of all cells oft he right rear optic thala-mus.“
	„Raising of all cells of the connection from the right rear optic thalamus to the left eye.“
	„Raising of all cells of the left eye.“
	„Raising of all areas of the brain and of the spinal cord which are connected to the left eye and these connections themselves.“
SEC	**Transmission:** like in **chapter 4.7.1.**
EXI	**Exit:** like in **chapter 4.8.**

Note 1: This alternative is suited very well for more obstinate cases.

Note 2: The said in alternative p1) in note 2 is valid also here.

Note 3: It is **generally** advantageous for the removal of a problem to strive for the good condition **with different methods.**

Note 4: The clairvoyant sees how all relevant areas are brought to brightness.

Note 5: You have already read in several examples above how to deal with the word „raising".

4.6.3.24. Alternative p4): To restore the vision (IV) in serious cases

Steps	Restoration
ENT	**Entry** like in example **ENT1 + ENT2**
FOC	**Focusing** like in example **FOC1 (F1-F5)**
CLE	**Cleaning** like in **chapter 4.4.3.**
DIA	**Diagnosis Steps** like in **chapter 4.5.3.**
RES-I	**Main Steps:**
R1	„Raising of all cells ..." like in alternative p3), **but...**
SEC	**Transmission:** like in **chapter 4.7.1.**
EXI	**Exit:** like in **chapter 4.8.**

Note 1: In serious cases the disturbed vision is usually based on strong violations of the divine order of the universe.

Note 2: Here the emotional-mental area <u>has to</u> be cleaned correctly, because there are strong negative information massiveness which can`t be dissolved satisfactorily even with alternative p3).

Note 3: And it shows that definitely the topics „arrogance" (among others to God), having criticism addiction, hate etc. play a big part in eye problems.

Note 4: The technology with the forefinger left is the basis, but it will be difficult without the centuries-old method about forgiveness, repentance and mercy. It isn`t about the improper excesses which some institutions have organized but about the inner confess.

Note 5: So here at first it is to proceed according to alternative 4.6.6.4 and only then according to alternative p3)!!!

Note 6: It is not recommended to correct such a serious problem without a clairvoyant! Please look for a reliable practioner with spiritual healing plus clairvoyants.

<u>Because:</u> You need the certainty that the negative causes are really dissolved.

Note 7: Please do not mistake a clairvoyant working in such way at the recovery area with e.g. a (channel-) medium.

4.6.3.25. Alternative q): Restoration of bipolar signals such as Parkinson, cancer

Steps	Restoration
ENT	**Entry** like in example **ENT1 + ENT2**
FOC	**Focusing** like in example **FOC1 (F1-F5)**
CLE	**Cleaning** like in **chapter 4.4.3.**
DIA	**Diagnosis Steps** like in **chapter 4.5.3.**
RES-I	**Main Steps:**
R1	„Restore all polarities to the norm of the Creator."
R2	„Restore all bipolar signals to the norm of the Creator."
R3	„I transfer the time for person XY to 10 p.m. And now I use the time 10 p.m. – 10.17 p.m."
R4	„,I concentrate on the **2 little fingers** of my hands."
R5	„I imagine a light **arc** betweeen the little fingers. Light arc, please."
R6	„The information of the <u>events</u> **streams from the left little finger** to the right little finger."
R7	„I feel into this light stream and concentrate on it."
R8	„Now I concentrate on the light arc, **simultaneously** to the second vertebra from below (in the coccyx) and also simultaneously to the events which triggered the illness 7-10 years ago."
R9	„I project the events so to speak in the light arc."
R10	„I wait and concentrate and with that I reduce the signals"
R11	„So I proceed until 10.17 p.m.."

R12	**Note:** From 10.17 p.m. on I turn the look further inside and hear into myself. When I feel that an information environment is coming towards me and an opinion arises within me, then I project at will a connecting line from the place of the environment to the light arc.
R13	„Restore all signals to the norm of the Creator."
SEC	**Transmission:** like in **chapter 4.7.1.**
EXI	**Exit:** like in **chapter 4.8.**

Note 1: If we hold our hands horizontal in front of us, then the light arc (= half a circle) of the open consciousness runs above the hands and the light arc (= half a circle) of the subconscious below the hands.

Note 2: We, so to speak, take signals from our aura surroundings and project these onto the light arc. 27)

Note 3: The colors give information about the scale from active (=red) to passive (= blue).

Note 4: The better we feel the sooner the signals will be reduced.

Note 5: At the same time this is a good method for the balance of the signals, e.g in case of Parkinson, cancer…

Note 6: We already reached the **first level of stabilization with R11.**

Note 7: By this complete action we change the negative information and the disturbed control. 28)

4.6.3.26. Alternative r): Information structure of the illness of an organ and also to delete the first 5 central cells by plasma glove 3)

Steps	Restoration
ENT	Entry like in example **ENT1 + ENT2**
FOC	**Focusing** like in example **FOC1 (F1-F5)**
CLE	**Cleaning** like in **chapter 4.4.3.**
DIA	**Diagnosis Steps** like in **chapter 4.5.3.**
RES-I	**Main Steps:**
R1	„I see the negative information abut the cell structure of the illness."
R2	„I cover my hand with a **glove of hot plasma.**"
R3	„Now I seize this negative **information massiveness** with the glove of hot plasma and lead it out of the 5m sphere of the consciousness to the macro- level into the silvery white cube for the transformation into divinely pure light."
R4	„Now I remove the **first 5 central cells** with the glove of hot plasma and lead them out to the macro-level into the silvery white cube for the transformation into divinely pure light."
R5	„Now I take 1 **cell** with living matter from the ultra-distant area and place this cell on the position which the first cell of disaster took before."
R6	„Then I take the next 4 cells out of the ultra-distant area and give them the order to lead the organ into the light step by step."
R7	„Restoration of all subordinate cells to the norm of the Creator."
R8	„Restore all connections of the organs and cells with each other and restore all controls by the pituitary. Perfect control of the organ by the pituitary."
SEC	**Transmission:** like in **chapter 4.7.1.**
EXI	**Exit:** like in **chapter 4.8.**

Note 1: The <u>information about the illness</u> is removed here, as well as in alternative u).

Note 2: Unlike to the alternative u), the information about the organ is not being changed here, but 5 cells are directly removed from the organ.

Note 3: This is possible, because these cells exist not only at the physical level but also at the astral and the mental level.

Note 4: It should be clear that we have to provide substitute cells at such a change to maintain the totality of the boody.

Note 5: Furthermore, is it also valid here that **with that procedure the cause of the illness at the emotional level is not solved yet.** Merely the information structure of the illness has been removed.

Note 6: If this cause <u>isn`t</u> dissolved according to note 5, then the problem is mildened only temporarily.

Note 7: And please take into account that the most of dissolving methods just seem to dissolve. (Please read to this the preface again.)

Note 8: The clairvoyant sees how the negative massiveness (= an intelligent structure) fights against its withdrawal. If the massiveness has crossed the 5m range, then increasing brightness appears.

Note 9: WARNING: Please never do this exercise without the plasma glove.

Note 10: WARNING: As a clairvoyant, **don`t go into** the event, but always look only from the side (flank).

4.6.3.27. Alternative s): Removal of cancer cells by sky perspective

Steps	Restoration
ENT	**Entry** like in example **ENT1 + ENT2**
FOC	**Focusing** like in example **FOC1 (F1-F5)**
CLE	**Cleaning** like in **chapter 4.4.3.**
DIA	**Diagnosis Steps** like in **chapter 4.5.3.**
RES-I	**Main Steps:**
R1	„I see the blue sky above my shoulders."
R2	„I put the cylinder on the ill organ. With that the removal of the ill cells starts (flying away at the information level).
R3	„There is no skin on the way of exit."
R4	„These cells are regenerated in the silvery white cube to the norm of the Creator."
SEC	**Transmission:** like in **chapter 4.7.1.**
EXI	**Exit:** like in **chapter 4.8.**

Note 1: It is particularly interesting that with this exercise **cancer cells** can be removed on information level. **And this applies also** to the negative **information** about the cell structure. And this thought process prevents that new negative information creeps in.

Note 2: We open the information channels with the approach of the sky perspective. The meaning of the removal of the information and the method is described by Grigori Grabovoi. [6]

Note 3: At first the approach looks complex, but it is really simple if you look at the graphic of Svetlana Smirnova[34]. Just imagine a bundle of parallel cylinders which is put vertically on the organ.

Note 4: Imagine the color of the <u>blue</u> sky above the shoulders.

Note 5: Please take into account the boundary conditions that the cylinders must'n overlap. And every cell needs its own cylinder.

Note 6: The clairvoyant sees how the cancer cells are flying through the cylinders to the outside. They often are really removed by suction.

Note 7: Please take into account that the removal of information is not the same as the removal of time.

4.6.3.28. Alternative t): Restoration by reference to the book "Practice of the Control" in case of cancer

Steps	Restoration
ENT	**Entry** like in example **ENT1 + ENT2**
FOC	**Focusing** like in example **FOC1 (F1-F5)**
CLE	**Cleaning** like in **chapter 4.4.3.**
DIA	**Diagnosis Steps** like in **chapter 4.5.3.**
RES-I	**Main Steps:**
R1	„Please, Christ hear me."
R2	„I ask for help for person XY."
R3	„I ask for the restoration of the lungs affected by cancer **analogously to the document** of the cure of Berischwili Iwan Georgijewitsch in 13.9.1993 and his application of the same day for Grigori Grabovoi, like it is denoted in the German translation „Praxis der Steuerung, volume 3", pages 109 – 171."
R4	„Please, Grigori Grabovoi hear me. Please support this process."
SEC	**Transmission:** like in **chapter 4.7.1.**
EXI	**Exit:** like in **chapter 4.8.**

Note 1: Of course, we have to find the data to **R3** in advance from the volumes 1-3 of "Praxis der Steuerung" (Practice of the Control).

Note 2: Please, pay attention that you refer clearly and obviously and don`t forget the date. In addition, we should quote all documents to the respective case. But quoting means not to read everything aloud. A quotation like in R3 is sufficient.

Note 3: There are **often several documents** to every case in the volumes "Praxis der Steuerung".

Note 4: Since all cases are witnessed notarially, we can refer to it to achieve the same effect on us.

Note 5: Please take into account that in all cases of the examples listed in the 3 volumes, it is not about copying the example, but about the cure method respectively applied there, even if the method isn`t mentioned in detail.

Example: So at an example about the dematerialization of a bottle it is not about the dematerialization of a bottle, but to use this method for the dematerialization of pollutants in the body.

Note 6: The clairvoyant sees how the pollutants leave the body: quite slowly!

4.6.3.29. Alternative u): Change of the information about an ill organ in the "area of the creative information"

Steps	Restoration
ENT	**Entry** like in example **ENT1 + ENT2**
FOC	**Focusing** like in example **FOC1 (F1-F5)**
CLE	**Cleaning** like in **chapter 4.4.3.**
DIA	**Diagnosis Steps** like in **chapter 4.5.3.**
RES-I	**Main Steps:**
R1	Note 1: The area of the creative information is described very well by Svetlana Smirnova. 2) And this area is described in detail by Grigori Grabovoi. 18)
	Note 2: If we work in the area of the creative information, then we are able to change the information which determines us (so to speak the movie of our life).
	Note 3: We work out from the soul and receive pictures in the consciousness.
	Note 4: If we change these pictures into the positive, then our situation also changes and also our physical reality, i.e. our body.
	Note 5: In this area of the creative information we can identify the area of e.g. an ill organ and then insert some new information for the organ.
	Note 6: Since at this method the macro-level is entered, the information of the illness is changed at the same time, too.

	Note 7: But please RESsider that behind every illness there is a cause (e.g. a shock, malposition of character etc.).
	Note 8: So we should dissolve 3 things: a) The negative information about the organ b) The negative information about the illness c) The negative information about the cause of the illness (e.g. according to alternative f) or according to 6.4.4.6.)
SEC	**Transmission:** like in **chapter 4.7.1.**
EXI	**Exit:** like in **chapter 4.8.**

4.6.3.30. Alternative v): Creating of a rescuer cell with a number sequence in it

Steps	Restoration
ENT	**Entry** like in example **ENT1 + ENT2**
FOC	**Focusing** like in example **FOC1 (F1-F5)**
CLE	**Cleaning** like in **chapter 4.4.3.**
DIA	**Diagnosis Steps** like in **chapter 4.5.3.**
RES-I	**Main Steps:**
R1	„I take a **light sphere** with living matter from the **ultra-distant** area to the forefinger right."
R2	„I fill this sphere with silvery white light."
R3	„I write the **word 'rescuer cell'** in it, give the '8' in addition and also the symbol of infinity (∞)."
R4	**„In addition, I insert the number sequence** for the illness 'XY'."
R5	„Now I let everything shine in bright violet light."
R6	„I lead this rescuer cell into the ill organ."
R7	**„Reproduction** of this cell **according to Fibonacci**, clockwise." + **Impulse**
SEC	**Transmission:** like in **chapter 4.7.1.**
EXI	**Exit:** like in **chapter 4.8.**

Note 1: The creation of rescuer cells is described very well by Svetlana Smirnova. 12)

Note 2: Preferentially take a cell from the ultra-distant area.

Note 3: After the placement of the rescue cell into the ill organ, give as a precaution the impulse for the reproduction of the rescuer cell according to the number sequence of Fibonacci (see to this note 4 in alternative p2).

Note 4: The use of the rescuer cell is a very important technology, especially in case of cancer.

Note 5: The clairvoyant sees the cell and then also its reproduction.

Note 6: To give the impulse in **R7 by forefinger right.**

Note 7: In case of serious illnesses it has to be worked in this way again and again until the organ is finally healthy.

4.6.3.31 Alternative w): Cube in cone in cube plus norm cell of the Creator for the restoration of cell level, blood and lymph

Steps	Restoration
ENT	**Entry** like in example **ENT1 + ENT2**
FOC	**Focusing** like in example **FOC1 (F1-F5)**
CLE	**Cleaning** like in **chapter 4.4.3.**
DIA	**Diagnosis Steps** like in **chapter 4.5.3.**
RES-I	**Main Steps:**
R1	**Note 1:** In the chapter „Cleaning", in the alternative h) the placing of the geometry without the rescuer cell is desribed.
	Note 2: The using of cube in cone in cube with a standardized rescuer cell is in this chapter **not only for the cleaning** of pressures, **but also for an increased healing** and the restoration of cells to the norm of the Creator.
	Note 3: Please note that this geometry should be placed into the aorta only about 10 cm behind the cardiac output.
	Note 4: Please take the formulations **C1-C5** from the chapter ‚Cleaning' and then add the rescuer cell to the geometry like shown in alternative v) R1-R6 for a sphere which is passed into the organ.
	Note 5: The clairvoyant sees how the condition of the blood cells improves. And the color appearance becomes much brighter and brighter.

	Note 6: The blood is a special juice! The body tries to keep every illness away from the blood as long as possible.
	Note 7: If an illness is already in the blood, then the highest urgency for regeneration is given.
	Note 8: In addition, this method is also very suitable for prevention. One time every 14 days is a good measure.
SEC	**Transmission:** like in **chapter 4.7.1.**
EXI	**Exit:** like in **chapter 4.8.**

4.6.3.32 Alternative x): Control of situations which are out of control (drugs, alcohol,...) as well as all other problems without progress

Ablauf-Schritte	(Wieder-)Herstellung
ENT	**Entry** like in example **ENT1 + ENT2**
FOC	**Focusing** like in example **FOC1 (F1-F5)**
CLE	**Cleaning** like in **chapter 4.4.3.**
DIA	**Diagnosis Steps** like in **chapter 4.5.3.**
RES-I	**Main Steps:**
R1	„I notice the coarse-grained system of person XY and search for the differentiations."
R2	„I slip **mentally with the hand** over the information of person XY and feel this granularity. I remodel it to the norm of the Creator."
R3	„Now **I remodel the input situation of the problem** (addiction...)."
R4	„For that I curl like into a carpet and roll into infinity to a point."
R5	„Now I transfer the time for person XY to 10.03 p.m. and concentrate on the 2 forefingers of my hands from 10.03 p.m. to 10.04 p.m."
R6	„**I switch the input source** of the (addiction) information into the source of the future positive information."
R7	„May person XY be free from his addiction and work, earn his money, etc."
SEC	**Transmission:** like in **chapter 4.7.1.**
EXI	**Exit: like in chapter 4.8.**

Note 1: If there is any knowledge about the situation, this knowledge can change the reality in advance. It helps to control. 33)

Note 2: Our perception with the senses is a control structure. And the perception by 3rd eye as well. If we notice something, we find something, then we start to control.

Note 3:. The input source of the (addiction) information of the affected person has to be exchanged by a norm information.

Thus: **The information which misdirects the person has to be exchanged.**

Note 4:. If we think faster than person XY who is out of the norm, then we are able to control effectively.

Note 5: For that we mentally go into infinity. There we are able to exchange this input source of the (addiction) information for a source of standard life (which is necessary).

Note 6: Do this exercise like that: 5 days, 1 day break, 5 days.

Note 7: „Addiction" is just an example and can be exchanged with any chosen problem.

Note 8: The affected person has to understand that his/her behaviour is not according to the norm.

4.6.3.33. Alternative y): Restoration of man from the most serious illness by concentration on a picture

Steps	Restoration
ENT	**Entry** like in example **ENT1 + ENT2**
FOC	**Focusing** like in example **FOC1 (F1-F5)**
CLE	**Cleaning** like in **chapter 4.4.3.**
DIA	**Diagnosis steps** like in **chapter 4.5.3.**
RES-I	**Main steps:**
R1	„I concentrate on the picture for the restoration of man from the most serious illness."
R2	„Now I let the picture take effect on soul, mind and body and ask for…" (e.g. restoration of all cells of my liver according to the norm of the Creator)
SEC	**Transmission:** like in **chapter 4.7.1.**
EXI	**Exit:** like in **chapter 4.8.**

Note 1: The **title** of the picture is **"Restoration of man from the most serious illness".** It works from the physical body up to the spiritual body.

Note 2: See chapter 4.1.3 e) for the picture contemplation.

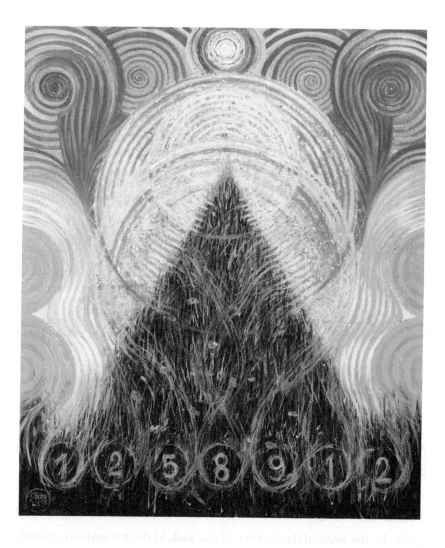

Artist: Sergey Jelezky, Öl auf Leinwand, 120x100cm, 2013

4.6.4. The partial Steps of the Restoration (Part II): The 6 Alternatives for the Control of Events (RES3)

Overview:

Alter-native	Aim	Methods of Restoration (shortcut: RES)
aa)	To produce events	Aim event by concentration on number ‚3‘
ab)	„ „	Control with the help of the number ‚8‘
ac)	„ „	Control with the help of sound waves
ad)	„ „	RES of events / conditions by concentration exercises for 31 days
ae)	„ „	Solution / harmonization of a situation by curved light column
af)	„ „	To realize an event by concentration on a picture (→ see **picture 4**).

Note 1: These exercises are oriented on producing an event or producing an aim attainment generally, not only in the health area.

Note 2: The variety makes it easy for us to be reminded again and again, by the normal day events, of our task of the permanent control.

Note 3: In the chapter 4.6.3 restoration (= part I) there are methods which make it able for us to work also on events.

Note 4: To keep the overview at such a variety, it is better not to use every method in all imagineable cases.

Note 5: In addition, with that we support the reaching of the routine within us. I.e. at a certain or similar question, we then automatically take a certain method due to the routine.

Note 6: At the desire that a general event (independent of any health question) may arise, the question of manipulation immediately comes up.

Note 7: It is right to strengthen the desire for an event that serves the aim "general rescue and harmonious development". We have to take care not to reduce the freedom of other persons by our actions.

Note 8: If another person pursues e.g. something bad, we can send love and harmony to him, but not the desire of him leaving his intention.

Note 9: If it is a machine which is destructive, we can work on having an effect on the "switching off", so that harmony arises.

Note 10: If we nevertheless try to manipulate, then our approach does not work or it will harm us, if not immediately, then later.

4.6.4.1 Alternative aa): Aim event by concentration on the number „3'

Steps	Restoration
ENT	**Entry** like in example **ENT1 + ENT2**
FOC	**Focusing** like in example **FOC1 (F1-F5)**
CLE	**Cleaning** like in **chapter 4.4.3.**
DIA	**Diagnosis steps** like in **chapter 4.5.3.**
RES-II	**Main steps:**
R1	**Note 1:** This method is also described very vell by Svetlana Smirnova [12].
	Note 2: It is important that we know exactly that there is a certain, desired future.
	Note 3: Here it is about <u>subsequent</u> events, the result which we want to achieve.
	Note 4: With that the concentration on **number „3'** at **simultaneous** thinking is suitable very well to fix the result of e.g. a medical, practical healing or spiritual healing treatment <u>before</u> the appointment: „After the session the patient may go home happily and relieved."
	Note 5: The clairvoyant sees a picture suitable for the issue. This number possibly comes from the Creator as a sign that the event has <u>matured</u>.
	Note 6: Sometimes a special sign appears which arises as a mixture of 3 and 5 to show that the event is completely initiated <u>and</u> matured.
	Note 7: At first this method seems very simple. But from the view of the logic of the universe, this method is of great importance. Therefore, Grigori Grabovoi repeats remembering our task to consider the subsequent events again and again.
SEC	**Transmission:** like in **chapter 4.7.1.**
EXI	**Exit:** like in **chapter 4.8.**

4.6.4.2 Alternative ab): Control of events with the help of <u>number „8'</u>

Steps	Restoration
ENT	**Entry** like in example **ENT1 + ENT2**
FOC	**Focusing** like in example **FOC1 (F1-F5)**
CLE	**Cleaning** like in **chapter 4.4.3.**
DIA	**Diagnosis steps** like in **chapter 4.5.3.**
RES-II	**Main steps:**
R1	**Note 1:** The exercise is described very well by Svetlana Smirnova. 12)
	Note 2: This exercise is good, because we make up our mind finally with one issue and set ourself in motion with that to cause events.
	Note 3: With the number „eight' it is then accomplished. Goethe already knew that in „witchcraft basics'. Please also take into account the differences between the upright and the lying eight . 17)+31)
	Note 4: Who knows the teaching of Grigori Grabovoi more exactly, learns that there is an own very productive number approach in the area of all plans beyond the health. **These number sequences run under the terms „business numbers". Those numbers are intended for all kinds of projects (i.e. business and private).**
	Note 5: Since we have a lot of good technologies for the causation of health anyway, we better should use this method with the eight for the procuring of accompanying circumstances.
	Note 6: Regardless to this, it is improtant to understand that almost any of the methods can and should always be used also at other areas.
SEC	**Transmission:** like in **chapter 4.7.1.**
EXI	**Exit:** like in **chapter 4.8.**

4.6.4.3 Alternative ac): Control of events with the help of <u>sound waves</u>, e.g the thyroid gland

Steps	Restoration
ENT	**Entry** like in example **ENT1 + ENT2**
FOC	**Focusing** like in example **FOC1 (F1-F5)**
CLE	**Cleaning** like in **chapter 4.4.3.**
DIA	**Diagnosis steps** like in **chapter 4.5.3.**
RES-II	**Main steps:**
R1	„Rescue and harmonious development for all and everyone."
R2	„Restoration of the norm of the Creator of all cells of my thyroid gland."
R3	„I connect this message with the sound noise ‚XZ' by thoughts."
SEC	**Transmission:** like in **chapter 4.7.1.**
EXI	**Exit:** like in **chapter 4.8.**

Note 1: This method is also well described by Svetlana Smirnova. [12]

Note 2: The really good with this method is that <u>everyday life is full of sound</u> from various sources and lasts almost nonstop.

Note 3: With that we are able to work on our goal realization almost constantly. With that we can reach the level of the procedure of „permanent control" recommended by Grigori Grabovoi.

Note 4: Please use each offered noise individually: once we work with the sound „X", then with the sound „Y". **That reinforces the effect.**

Note 5: Please note the right sequence: ask for others first and then for yourself, otherwise it won`t succeed. Please read to that in Grigori Grabovoi „Rescue and harmonious Development". 29).

Note 6: The sound goes to infinity. Consequently, the clairvoyant sees so-called standing waves, e.g. running into infinity or also the cosmos into which the transferred information of the sound is moving on.

Note 7: The recovery of the thyroid gland is selected here as event. But we can put any event here.

4.6.4.4 Alternative ad): Restoration of events/ conditions by concentration exercises (over 31 days)

Steps	Restoration
ENT	**Entry** like in example **ENT1 + ENT2**
FOC	**Focusing** like in example **FOC1 (F1-F5)**
CLE	**Cleaning** like in **chapter 4.4.3.**
DIA	**Diagnosis steps** like in **chapter 4.5.3.**
RES-II	**Main steps:**
R1	**Note:** The **31-days-exercises** 16) have several advantages:
	1. If we have started with it once, then we want to continue. That keeps us on track.
	2. The text is as difficult in Russian as in the German and English translation. The difficulty is not the language, but our understanding.
	3. Consciously reading of these texts again and again, there opens then a consciousness windows with increasing time so that the text becomes more understandable. **Grigori Grabovoi has installed key texts in these exercises which cause this opening by the time. Everything depends on our personal development.** It doesn't help, if we refer to have been spiritualist for 20 years to get a preferred opening.
	4. We repeatedly synchronize ourselves with these number exercises to the rythm of the cosmos.
	5. On the 29th day of every month we reach a higher **spiritual** state.

	6. **Since we are able to give our individual wishes into every exercise, we permanently get on**
	Thus: These exercises should be „daily standard" for everyone.
	7. As long as we are able to keep our mind busy with this „true event", we can`t want, think, feel and act wrong.
SEC	**Transmission:** like in **chapter 4.7.1.**
EXI	**Exit:** like in **chapter 4.8.**

4.6.4.5 Alternative ae): Harmonization/ solution of a situation by bent light column

Steps	Restoration
ENT	**Entry** like in example **ENT1 + ENT2**
FOC	**Focusing** like in example **FOC1 (F1-F5)**
CLE	**Cleaning** like in **chapter 4.4.3.**
DIA	**Diagnosis steps** like in **chapter 4.5.3.**
RES-II	**Main steps:**
R1	„I see the **light column** of the Creator in front of myself approx. 50 cm vertically."
R2	„General rescue and harmonious development."
R3	„I imagine the event which I want to reach."
R4	„I put this information mentally into the light column of the Creator."
R5	**„Now I bend the light column to a bow so that the center of my information flows to the highest point of the curvature."**
R6	**„I hold on the information at this point and concentrate on it."**
R7	„And now I let go the bow."
R8	„The bow becomes a light column again and my desired event is catapulted to the macro-sphere."
SEC	**Transmission:** like in **chapter 4.7.1.**
EXI	**Exit:** like in **chapter 4.8.**

Note 1: The method is shown very well graphically by Svetl

12) A bow, like "arrow and bow".

Note 2: With this method the information gets like a flash to level where it provides the putting into action into the earthly reality.

Note 3: It doesn`t mean yet that the event also arrives like a flash. Only the divine level knows when the right time is.

Note 4: The clairvoyant sees e.g. the desire like a white cloud which is soaked up in the center. Then the information suddenly leaves the geometry into the direction of the cosmos.

Alternative af): <u>To realize an event</u> by concentration on a picture

Steps	Restoration
ENT	**Entry** like in example **ENT1 + ENT2**
FOC	**Focusing** like in example **FOC1 (F1-F5)**
CLE	**Cleaning** like in **chapter 4.4.3.**
DIA	**Diagnosis steps** like in **chapter 4.5.3.**
RES-II	**Main steps:**
R1	„I concentrate on the picture for the realization of an event."
R2	„Now I let the picture take effect on soul, mind and body and ask for…" (e.g. passing my final exams, so I am able to do more for the development of society.).
SEC	**Transmission:** like in **chapter 4.7.1.**
EXI	**Exit:** like in **chapter 4.8.**

Note 1: The **title** of the picture is **"To realize an event".**

Note 2: See chapter 4.1.3 e) to the picture contemplation.

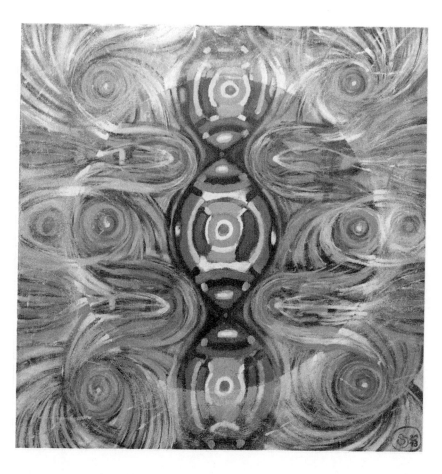

Künstler: Sergey Jelezky, Öl auf lwd, 80x80cm, 2013

4.6.5. The partial Steps of the Restoration (Part III): 8 Alternatives with special Solutions (RES4)

Overview:

Alter-native	Aim	Methods of the Restoration (shortcut: RES)
ba)	Solution for a particular purpose	Perception of white light at night
bb)	„ „	Allround-method with 2 light columns, e.g. to eliminate disharmonies or to aquire an ability
bc)	„ „	To „wiretap" knowledge
bd)	„ „	To bring an organ to the norm by **rainbow** concentration
be)	„ „	Quick search of resort by ball on head and in front of the root of the nose
bf)	„ „	To make my reality eternal
bg)	„ „	Special dealing with numbers for psychological standardization
bh)	„ „	To achieve the aim by self-defined number sequences

Note 1: These special solutions usually aim to a particular event or condition to come up (like in chapter 4.6.4,), but these methods in this chapter do also have another character.

Note 2: If these methods wouldn't be presented in a seperate chapter, then they could easily be overlooked completely wrongly in the variety of methods.

Note 3: Each of the following methods have a special advantage. An example: The "perception of the white light at night" works for us 8 hours in the right direction at 8 hours of sleep. It's not easy to perform to practice 8 hours a day.

Note 4: So the other exercises of this chapter also have something special.

Note 5: It is advisable to look at each of these exercises accurately.

Note 6: It becomes very exciting when we are able to define number sequences by ourselves, like the example of alternative bh) shows.

4.6.5.1 Alternative ba): Perception of the white light at night

Steps	Restoration
ENT	**Entry** like in example **ENT1 + ENT2**
FOC	**Focusing** like in example **FOC1 (F1-F5)**
CLE	**Cleaning like in chapter 4.4.3.**
DIA	**Diagnosis steps like in chapter 4.5.3.**
RES-III	**Main steps:**
R1	„**Concentration on the right earlobe and the organ „X"** <u>at the same time</u>**."**
R2	„**I adjust to the absorption of the white light tonight with all cells of the organ „X" for the restoration of all cells of the organ „X" according to the norm of the Creator."**
SEC	**Transmission: like in chapter 4.7.1.**
EXI	**Exit: like in chapter 4.8.**

Note 1: We will find the information to this issue by Grigori Grabovoi[6] (and there in chapter 4) and with Svetlana Smirnova. [12]

Note 2: This method stops the process and removes the source of fast going swelling processes.

Note 3: And that mostly lasts for 8 hours long by subconscious. With which other method do we work so intensively otherwise?

Note 4: This method is to put on before sleep in the evening every day and it is a blessing.

Note 5: Fast processes require a permanent diagnosis and correction.

Note 6: This method, of course, is also possible for other illness processes than the swelling and often provides fast results.

Note 7: The clairvoyant would have to watch a sleeping person to see something.

Note 8: <u>Here is also valid:</u> This exercise always works, even if we can't see anything with the 3rd eye.

4.6.5.2 Alternative bb): Allround-method e.g. to remove disharmonies or e.g. to acquire an ability by color concentration with 3 light columns

Steps	Restoration
ENT	**Entry** like in example **ENT1 + ENT2**
FOC	**Focusing** like in example **FOC1 (F1-F5)**
CLE	**Cleaning** like in **chapter 4.4.3.**
DIA	**Diagnosis steps** like in **chapter 4.5.3.**
RES-III	**Main steps:**
R1	„I see a vertical, silvery white light column on the <u>left</u> of myself."
R2	„I connect this light column with the teaching of the „general rescue and harmonious development" by Grigori Grabovoi."
R3	„A second light column with the color Y is on the <u>right</u> of me."
R4	**„I put the desired event "Z" into this 2nd light column."**
R5	**„The event shall occur up to…" (Date!)**
R6	„The light of the 2 columns rises up to the infinity and merges there."
R7	„A new light beam forms which contains a mixed light out of the 2 colors and flows through me centrally from above."
R8	**„This light spreads in the whole surrounding and also solves the problems of all others."**
R9	„I recognize that I permanently shall pass on this knowledge for the solution of problems."
R10	„<u>In addition</u>, I now give this task of passing on into the light column at the right of my side."
SEC	**Transmission:** like in **chapter 4.7.1.**
EXI	**Exit:** like in **chapter 4.8.**

Note 1: The right light column shall be any bright color (gold, lilac, pink).

Note 2: The desired event could be e.g. the recovery of the **organ** "YY" or the **ability** "ZZ" etc.

Note 3: This exercise of Grigori Grabovoi is well shown by Svetlana Smirnova. 12)

Note 4: The exercise has to be done best repeatedly at the time between 10 p.m. and 11 p.m. at local time.

Note 5: The clairvoyant sees not only the light particles of the emerging beam from above, but also for example a picture to the task of passing on to others or a picture to the condition arising in us.

Note 6: Read also to this Note 10 in chapter 4.6.6.1 about the effect of the teachings of Grigori Grabovoi.

4.6.5.3 Alternative bc): To "wiretap" knowledge

Steps	Restoration
ENT	**Entry** like in example **ENT1 + ENT2**
FOC	**Focusing** like in example **FOC1 (F1-F5)**
CLE	**Cleaning** like in **chapter 4.4.3.**
DIA	**Diagnosis steps** like in **chapter 4.5.3.**
RES-III	**Main steps:**
R1	„I transform my time to 10 p.m. local time."
R2	„I **activate** all lectures of Grigori Grabovoi which he adjusted into the Akasha."
R3	„Now I load the knowledge, deposited by Grigori Grabovoi, to the issue ,Healing in the topic XY`."
R4	„Grigori Grabovoi, please help."
R5	„Transfer this knowledge to me."
SEC	**Transmission:** like in **chapter 4.7.1.**
EXI	**Exit:** like in **chapter 4.8.**

Note 1: Grigori Grabovoi has held approx. 200 lectures and deposited all lectures in the spiritual area (Akasha chronics).

Note 2: Sometimes the problem, for which we are looking for the solution, dissolves at once.

Note 3: Maybe you are wondering whether your issue is deposited by Grigori Grabovoi at all? It is better you just try it. <u>Because:</u> 200 topics

are a very wide spectrum.

Note 4: Fewest people have more than 10 areas of interests for which they really want to get new information.

Note 5: The deposited issues concern all possible areas (e.g. crystals etc.), not only for recovery.

Note 6: The clairvoyant sees at the call for activation, e.g. a book, which swells up suddenly. And at the transfer of knowledge, e.g. letters could tumble down.

Note 7: If we name the issue, then information will be sent to us by the one or other way.

4.6.5.4. Alternative bd): To bring organs to the norm by rainbow

Steps	Restoration
ENT	**Entry** like in example **ENT1 + ENT2**
FOC	**Focusing** like in example **FOC1 (F1-F5)**
CLE	**Cleaning** like in **chapter 4.4.3.**
DIA	**Diagnosis steps** like in **chapter 4.5.3.**
RES-III	**Main steps:**
R1	„I imagine the colors of the rainbow, **starting with red.**"
R2	„I will conduct these colors of the rainbow through myself one after the other."
R3	„If one color holds me tighter than the other ones, then I concentrate on it particularly."
R4	„Now I start with the color red."
SEC	**Transmission:** like in **chapter 4.7.1.**
EXI	**Exit:** like in **chapter 4.8.**

Note 1: We have to keep up concentration for 5 minutes on this color which holds me tight.

Note 2: This exercise is very effective.

Note 3: Who can`t see the color in front of the 3rd eye, can go through the rainbow colors by thoughts nevertheless.

Note 4: The clairvoyant sees the color which another person arranges

by thoughts. I.e. the colors develop, even if we <u>can`t</u> see them by ourselves.

Note 5: Temporarily the non-clairvoyant can be lead by his feeling to a color.

Note 6: If there is neither the view nor the feeling to a color, so the mental "pushing through" of the rainbow colors is still effective and harmonizing.

Note 7: The color methods have charm, since colors automatically lead into infinity and connect us with it.

Note 8: The rainbow in the sky does not only cause joy within us again and again, but also attracts many people really magically. This becomes understandable when we think about the influence of this color spectrum onto our soul.

4.6.5.5 Alternative be): Fast searching of resort by ball on head and in front of the root of the nose

Steps	Restoration
ENT	**Entry** like in example **ENT1 + ENT2**
FOC	**Focusing** like in example **FOC1 (F1-F5)**
CLE	**Cleaning** like in **chapter 4.4.3.**
DIA	**Diagnosis steps** like in **chapter 4.5.3.**
RES-III	**Main steps:**
R1	„I see the problem „XY" 2 cm in front of my forehead in a sphere with the radius of 1 cm on the height of the 3rd eye."
R2	„Now I connect the sphere with the first segment of the upper information center (above my head) with 2 beams which mark the segment."
SEC	**Transmission:** like in **chapter 4.7.1.**
EXI	**Exit:** like in **chapter 4.8.**

Note 1: This method is shown graphically well by Svetlana Smirnova. [13]

Note 2: The segment which contains the solution is in the sphere above the head and points towards the nose.

Note 3: This method causes the solution relatively quick. The solution comes by thoughts or by a suitable picture or by a situation in which we recognize what we have to do.

Note 4: The divine level knows exactly in what kind of form we are able to understand something.

Note 5: And if there is a person near to us who is able to receive messages, then the information sometimes comes in that form in which the person is able to receive it, but the person does not necessarily understand it.

Note 6: Of course, the clairvoyant sees the mental construction. If an isosceles white cross appears in front of the sphere in addition, then he knows that the issue comes into balance.

Note 7: This method should not be misused for disposing of every little problem to the Creator. On the other hand in most cases it is better to ask for help from "above" rather than to struggle. The right balance is necessary.

Note 8: It is good, if we already opted out of the events before asking for a solution.

4.6.5.6 Altenative bf): To make my reality <u>eternal</u>

Steps	Restoration
ENT	**Entry** like in example **ENT1 + ENT2**
FOC	**Focusing** like in example **FOC1 (F1-F5)**
CLE	**Cleaning** like in **chapter 4.4.3.**
DIA	**Diagnosis steps** like in **chapter 4.5.3.**
RES-III	**Main steps:**
R1	„I think of the property ‚X' which is imperfect for me."
R2	„But now I know that I have this property forever and in perfection beyond our reality."
R3	„There I am eternal."
R4	„888 898 1 2"
R5	„‚3' + I understand that there is an information area with which I can make my reality forever."
SEC	**Transmission:** like in **chapter 4.7.1.**
EXI	**Exit:** like in **chapter 4.8.**

Note 1: "The reality of eternity has its origin in man and vice versa the eternity of the environment contribute to the human knowledge of man's eternity." 26)

Note 2: At the restoration of man by number sequences by concentration, we change the world into the direction of eternal development, i.e. also us.

194

Note 3: I.e. **we open our originally eternal nature** which is capable to create the eternal body.

Note 4: <u>Thus:</u> This exercise opens us. If once we have understood this correctly, then we don`t need this exercise any more.

Note 5: In **R1** we think of something, i.e. we perceive.

Note 6: The ‚**3**‘ in **R5** is to see in continuation to ‚1‘ and ‚2‘ in **R4.** But the ‚3‘ has to be used a little bit differently.

Note 7: In **R5** we should understand what is said in **R5** and **simultaneously** think at ‚3‘.

Note 8: The method shown here is only one of the possibilities to make our reality eternal.

4.6.5.7 Alternative bg): Healing of a psychological condition with the use of e.g. the light sensibility of the eye and order of non-dying

Steps	Restoration
ENT	**Entry** like in example **ENT1 + ENT2**
FOC	**Focusing** like in example **FOC1 (F1-F5)**
CLE	**Cleaning** like in **chapter 4.4.3.**
DIA	**Diagnosis steps** like in **chapter 4.5.3.**
RES-III	**Main steps:**
R1	„I take the number sequence '**588 061 989 711**', which stands for the psychological state of the vision which has to be healed."
R2	„Now I fit in **after** this number sequence ,319' and the numbers of year, month and day, thus '58...711 319 20131224."
R3	„Now I place before the number sequence of the **light sensibility** of my eyes the following numbers and letters : 8889 ONE NINE. **Thus: 8889 ONE NINE 519 317 818 266.**"
SEC	**Transmission:** like in **chapter 4.7.1.**
EXI	**Exit:** like in **chapter 4.8.**

Note 1: You will find the complete number sequence for vision in **R1 + R2** in the "psycho"-numbers. 26)

Note 2: There are further, very interesting types of number dealing in the book „Number sequences of psychological Standardization".

Note 3: Of course, vision is a physical process. But if it is impaired, then the question about the psychological aspects arises which are responsible for that. In any case these causes are correctable.

Note 4: According to **chapter 4.6.6.4** the correction of heavy problems is a strong help beside the psycho numbers.

Note 5: The mixed sequence of numbers and letters in **R3** points out that there is a letter system besides the number system.

Note 6: The word „ONE" is to speak like that and we also have to imagine this like that.

Note 7: The „non-dying" has different approaches, depending on the terms world, so it has to be handled differently with economic terms than in case of psychological terms. [36]

Note 8: We will also find the number for the light sensibility in the „psycho"-numbers.

Note 9: In **R1 + R2** the vision problem is healed. In **R3** a „psycho"-number is used to arrange our non-dying. So in this exercise two very different processes in the issue „eyes" are connected with each other.

4.6.5.8 Alternative bh): Change of character by self-defined number sequence

Steps	Restoration
ENT	**Entry** like in example **ENT1 + ENT2**
FOC	**Focusing** like in example **FOC1 (F1-F5)**
CLE	**Cleaning** like in **chapter 4.4.3.**
DIA	**Diagnosis steps** like in **chapter 4.5.3.**
RES-III	**Main steps:**
R1	„By the now following number sequence I want to achieve more love in me."
R2	„I will notice at some point while reading that my perception by numbers works as it usually does by consciousness."
R3	„At that moment I will direct my consciousness to the sphere of realization of love."
R4	„I place the number sequence and read slowly **5216480171290829319814215 9871249**."
SEC	**Transmission:** like in **chapter 4.7.1.**
EXI	**Exit:** like in **chapter 4.8.**

Note 1: For each letter there is an 8-digit number sequence by Grigori Grabovoi. [26)]

Note 2: These number sequences to represent a letter are valid for every language.

Note 3: This makes it possible to express each word in form of a number sequence.

198

Note 4: At a 4-letter-word like „love" that is already 32 digits. You will wonder who shall work with that without any problems? But this is easier than you think. You just have to read the digits slowly and calmly.

Note 5: So in this exercise we can cause our aim of character purification by the combination of psychology and the principles of eternal development. And we can build up our personality aim-orientedly. **What a brilliant undertaking.**

Note 6: It is clear that we need the respective assignment of the number sequences to the sounds of a language. The number sequences can be found in the psycho-numbers. 26)

Note 7: You are free in the choice of the term, such as „love".

4.6.6. Complex Restorations (Part IV) – RES5

Overwiev:

Alter-native	Aim	Complex restoration
ca)	To build an ability	→ with 18 different methods
cb)	The complexity of a seemingly simple sub-ject	At the examples: - toothache - marital problems
cc)	An own space/time area	To create and use of a space/time area for the acquisition of an ability
cd)	Correction of heavy problems from mis-takes	By forgiveness and repentance…
ce)	Perfection	‚To be in paradise' by concentrati-on on a picture (→ see **picture 5**)

4.6.6.1 Alternative ca): To build an ability with <u>different</u> methods, e.g. 18 alternatives for the attainment of clairvoyance

A) <u>Notes</u>:

Note 1: You won`t find <u>any new</u> methods here.

Note 2: It is shown how you can e.g systematically build a new ability for yourself with <u>different</u> methods.

Note 3: Here it matters to use the circumstances, spread over a day, which are very different in the course of a day.

Note 4: Depending on the ability, the one or other method will accrue or will be omitted.

Note 5: Please consider that the attainment of the ability of clairvoyance is a mercy of God. With growing personality it will be given to everybody.

Note 6: Who attains or wants to attain this gift by „forced opening", usually gets a heavy damage in his health. The palette of problems then reaches from permanent headache to a tumor in the head, e.g. on the spot where the 3rd eye opens normally. Unreasonable people eventually risk to be withdrawn from life completely.

Note 7: The Creator knows who needs this gift. It also can be given for example so that people who are trained less spiritually can realize that there is a world beyond. Conversely, very spiritual people can be „slowed down" downright so that they give up their arrogance in the

first place.

Note 8: .. There are also other reasons why the Creator provides the one or other way for us. **We should never forget who is our Lord.**

Note 9: These methods are all helpful to us. But who attempts to achieve his aim by force, already harms 2 laws:

He puts his own efforts over the love of God.

He disturbs the harmony.

Note 10: How about the ability „to perfectly understand the teachings of Grigori Grabovoi"? Use for example the number for the teachings of Grigori Grabovoi of the „**General rescue, harmonious development and prevention of global catastrophes": 1784121**

The clairvoyant then sees e.g. the gorgeous cycle of a peacock or the oversized growing of a flower's pollen bag. Both images speak for themselves.

4.6.6.1 B) To build an ability with 18 different methods

	Approach to the method	Source
1	To place the **number for the psychological standardization** to this ability.	Bibliography 26)
2	To place numbers like e.g.: * To make the impossible possible * To reach the unreachable * To acquire new abilities * Expansion of knowledge in any area * Constant focus on the result * Correction of past events * Consequences of the corrrection of the past for present and future	The boook ‚Numbers for a successful Business' 30)
3	To place a new **principle** by ball.	Alternative g) in chapter 4.6.2.
4	Concentration exercise of the day + your wish to be held more than 5 seconds.	Bibliography 16) + Alternative ad) in chapter 4.6.4.
5	Request direct to God	
6	Ball above head and in front of the root of the nose.	Chapter 4.6.5.5.
7	To pursue the time axis to infinity when thinking about the issue.	Bibliography 24)
8	To give love in this issue again and again. To proceed similarly as in „love for the past, present and future".	Chapter 4.4.3.6.
9	Dissolving of all negative massiveness which slow us down at this issue.	Chapter 4.6.6.4.
10	To take an example from ‚Practice of the Control'.	Chapter 4.6.2. alternative i1)
11	By raising analogoulys to an ability	Chapter 4.6.3. alternative d1)
12	By ‚System of Education'	Chapter 4.6.3.9.

13	Mental connection with sound events and simultaneiously concentrating on your desired ability.	Chapter 4.6.4. alternative ac)
14	To create a space/time area and to fill it with this desired property.	Chapter 4.6.6.3.
15	Concentration on number ‚3‘	Chapter 4.6.4.1.
16	Concentration on number ‚8‘	Chapter 4.6.4.2.
17	By curved light column	Chapter 4.6.4.5.
18	By color concentration	Chapter 4.6.5.2.

4.6.6.2 Alternative cb): The complexity in an <u>apparantly</u> simple issue

Notes:

Note 1: Alternative a) in chapter 4.6.3.1 already offers an example to that, because there already are 2 methods connected with each other. In that example it is about to work both over the process of the illness (= numbers from „Restoration of the human Organism by Concentration on Numbers") and over the „Restoration of the Matter of Man by Concentration on Numbers".

The importance of the difference is only understood by those one who have attentively worked out the new conception of the world. 31)

<u>Because</u>: It is important to distinguish between the organism (which is just not the matter) and the matter.

Note 2: Let`s take the example „**toothache**". People have difficulties to recognize the real damaged spot. Maybe there are already some of our different body systems involved. Does the cause lie in the nerve of the tooth? Or does the cause lie e.g. in the lower jaw? And in the lower jaw area is it a question of gums, the oral mucosa, the 3rd branch of the trigeminal nerve or another nerve? Or is it a question of the lymphatic system? Etc. In addition, the question arises whether the cause may be at a completely different place due to the holistic construction of man? 31)

Note 3: If we look at a **marriage problem,** then the complexity also lets itself be seen, only the questions are different. Is it due to the aggressiveness of the one or to the claim of perfectionism of the other? Etc. There is a very

long list of psycho-number sequences for the changing work of character.
26)

Note 4: So there are a lot of good reasons why we often should work with a variety of <u>number sequences</u> from <u>different</u> areas.

Note 5: If the numbers really become too many, then the construction of an own space/time area for such an issue is helpful. This saves time. (See to that chapter 4.6.6.3)

Note 6: So on the one hand we have the possibility to use a variety of methods for an issue (like shown in chapter 4.6.6.1 at the example of the construction of an ability). On the other hand we have the possibility to optimally use the variety of the number sequences.

4.6.6.3 Alternative cc): An own space/time area

A) The <u>use</u> of an <u>own</u> space/time area

Notes:

Note 1: The construction of a self-defined space/time area is mentioned as a possibility by Grigori Grabovoi [24].

Note 2: Hugin Munin [25] has already mentioned the practical transfer in the context of the business numbers.

Note 3: An own space/time area created for a self-chosen issue can help to save much time, e.g. if we have a lot of number sequences.

Note 4: <u>Many</u> number sequences are the result of different points of view:

a) E.g. concerning the **control of a <u>project,</u>** because there we use the variety of the terms.
b) We also can enter **all numbers of an issue,** e.g. all number sequences for the musculature or the psycho-numbers into a space/time area.

c) Many number sequences incur e.g. when we want to work on a seemingly simple „**issue**" of a local illness in the body, in case of **working in different body systems.**

<u>Thus:</u> E.g. it is necessary to work on the toothache with the numbers of the dermal tissue, the numbers of the bone (jaw!), the numbers of the nerves in the jaw and in the tooth etc.

Note 5: Is the area created once, we can pay a „**short visit**" to this area on and off, to let this variety of terms and number sequences take an effect on us.

Note 6: Such a space/time area can, of course, also be created for many other applications.

An example: The creation of a complex geometry. If the process takes too long to be created with one session, we can start it in a space/time area and complete this construction with every visit to this area.

4.6.6.3 B) The creation of an own space/time area at the example of obtaining the ability of „intuition"

Steps	Restoration
ENT	**Entry** like in example **ENT1 + ENT2**
FOC	**Focusing** like in example **FOC1 (F1-F5)**
CLE	**Cleaning** like in **chapter 4.4.3.**
RES-IV	**Main steps:**
R1	„Christ, please help."
R2	„I take a space/time **point** and and pull the milieu in this point mentally apart to a space/time **area**."
R3	„Now I form the contour of man according to Leonardo Da Vinci`s design of man, at first 2-dimensionally, then 3-dimensionally, as a cavity."
R4	„I give to this **area**: Love (+impulse), harmony (+impulse), happiness (+impulse) and joy of the infinite eternal further development (+ impulse)."
R5	**„This is the area where the term ‚structure' coincides with the term ‚property'."**
R6	„The space/time area has the **name ‚Intuit'**."
R7	„In this space/time area the entering person shall get the following influences: Intuition 489611 094 892 Dimension of consciousness 1888888 9 1 Correct processing of the information 5555555 etc."
R8	**„Light sphere**, please, in front of the forefinger right."
R9	„I place the impulses in the light sphere Golden light, love, harmony, happiness and joy of the infinite eternal further development."
R10	**„Copy** of the light sphere, please."
R11	„This copy gets the task to wrap around the space/time area to protect the area from all negative influences."
R12	„Effective from now on until eternity."
R13	„Transfer around the space/time area." + Impulse.

R14	„The **original sphere** gets the task to monitor the functioning of the copy for all eternity."
SEC4	„Light connection, please, in front of the **forefinger right** to the **little finger of the right hand.**"
SEC6	„„„I pull the **original light sphere** from the **forefinger right to the right side up to the little finger of the right hand** and transmit it to infinity for the eternal further development."
SEC3	„Hamburg, 5.30 p.m. of summer time, 15.7.2013" + Impulse
SEC1	„Light connection, please, from the **forefinger left** to the little finger of the right hand."
SEC2	„I pull the scenario from the forefinger left **to the right side up to the little finger of the right hand** and transmit it to infinity for the eternal further development."
SEC3	„Place, date, time." + Impulse
EXI	**Exit:** like in example **chapter 4.8.**

Note 1: Grigori Grabovoi mentions the construction of an own space/time area. [24]

Note 2: An area is uniquely located by the intersection of two terms. The use of two terms determines the spatial coordinates.

Note 3: In **R7** it matters to deposit preferably all relevant terms plus number sequence of an issue. These terms and number sequences represent the content of the space/time area.

Note 4: The area has to be saved from negative influences, e.g. like in **R8-R11.**

Note 5: As long as we don`t inform other people about the coordinates and the name of the area, the area cannot be misused by anybody.

Note 6: If the space/time area is cleaned and protected, then only the creator of this area brings in the negative which he carries within himself.

Note 7: Although the use of a space/time area by several persons is possible, it has the disadvantage that every person who enters the area could also change the area.

Note 8: This influencing control can`t be prevented either, since we would violate against the freedom of others with such an application. Such a request of us would fall back on us negatively.

Note 9: If immutability is desired, then we keep the coordinates and the name of the area better to us.

Note 10: The clairvoyant sees e.g. how the protection for the area builds up which is installed in **R8-R11.**

Note 11: If an already created area shall be completed or changed afterwards, then the area has to be entered duly. See chapter 4.6.6.3 c) to this.

Note 12: Since we have worked at the right hand, the securing of the „placed" takes place differently here, compared to the most other exercises. The circumstance that „**SEC3**" takes place after „**SEC6**" has its correctness.

Note 13: And please don`t forget the proper exit in the end.

Note 14: Who worked with the space/time area once, will not want to miss it again, because the advantages overbalance by far the effort for the construction.

Note 15: The simultaneous processing of many terms has not only the charm of time saving, but also of the broad effect.

Note 16: The clairvoyant sees how this aura generally improves from visit to visit.

4.6.6.3 C) The entering of an already constructed space/time area

Steps	Restoration
ENT	**Entry** like in example **ENT1 + ENT2**
FOC	**Focusing** like in example **FOC1 (F1-F5)**
CLE	**Cleaning** like in **chapter 4.4.3.**
RES-IV	**Main steps:**
R1	„Christ, please help."
R2	„I call up the space/time area with the **name ‚Intuit'.**"
R3	„This is the space/time area where the term „structure" coincides with the term „property"."
R4	„Now I enter the space/time area with the name ‚Intuit'."
R5	„Activation of all terms and the matching number sequences for person „XY"."
R6	„Christ, please give light onto this number sequences so that the optimal effect in person „XY" can be obtained."
R7	„The materializing takes place in front of the background of the soul of the Creator."
R8	„Restoration of the norm of the Creator according to the prototype of the Creator in the topic „intuition"."
SEC	**Transmission:** like in **chapter 4.7.1.**
EXI	**Exit:** like in **chapter 4.8.**

4.6.6.4 Alternative cd): Correction of heavy problems or loads from mistakes (no matter whether in earlier lives (karma) or in this life) by elimination of the cause

Steps	Restoration
ENT	**Entry** like in example **ENT1 + ENT2**
FOC	**Focusing** like in example **FOC1 (F1-F5)**
CLE	**Cleaning** like in **chapter 4.4.3.**
RES-V	**Main steps:**
R1	„I go on the time axis of person „XY" to the time 5 years before birth."
R2	„I load into the light sphere in front of the forefinger left the issue „Arrogance towards God".
R3	„Christ, pleaase help to clear the relationship of person „XY" in this issue."
R4	„I decide to leave all events and experiences which are connected to the issue „**Arrogance**" and to having placed this issue above the love for God."
R5	„All persons involved have gone their way to the Creator, the events have gone their own way and I have gone my way to the Creator. All our ways have not crossed each other."
R6	„Heavenly Father, I ask for **forgiveness** that I placed this issue above the love for God."
R7	„And I ask for forgiveness that I placed this issue above the love for God also on the part of my ancestors."
R8	„Venerable Father, I ask for help and for the elimination of all aggressions which arised from that."
R9	„And I ask for the **dissolving** of all dependences of earthly desires which have arisen out of it."
R10	„And I ask for the **removal** of my adherence to a happy style of life which is the result of it. So please remove my sympathies and antipathies to everything, e.g. to my ideas or to my clinging or rejecting of other people."
R11	„Venerable Father, I **regret** that I have put this dependence over the love for God."

R12	„And I **regret** that I have passed on this dependence to my descendants and people close to me, possibly via many generations."
R13	„And I regret that I have not accepted all the possibilities of purification and catharsis that came to me in form of defeats, humiliations and the like across my road."
R14	„In fact, I myself have reacted with contempt and criticism of others."
R15	„And I have also loaded this non-acceptance of purification and catharsis on the shoulders of the before mentioned souls."
R16	**„So know I kneel in front of you, heavenly Father, at first slowly understanding that there is a divine order to which I also have to keep."**
R17	„Heavenly Father, I ask for forgiveness and mercy."
R18	„And so that all parties can easily go into the light, I`m now sending to all persons involved my love, first of all to you, heavenly Father. Then to all other persons involved."
SEC	**Transmission:** like in **chapter 4.7.1.**
EXI	**Exit:** like in **chapter 4.8.**

Note 1: This procedure is not advisable without a clairvoyant, since most people do not have the necessary deep religious fervor any more.

And the examination of the situation by clairvoyance after the apology is a crucial litmus test which provides feedback directly.

The visit to a medium is not a substitute for this procedure. Please consult a competent center which has the competence and not just promises it.

Note 2: This method does nothing without a deep, inner fervor, because then God won`t let us „out".

Note 3: The sheer variety of steps shows the importance of this method.

Note 4: We can dissolve burdens/problems with <u>this</u> way which cannot be done by other methods of dissolutions. They only seem to be sucessful.

Note 5: Deap-seated stresses with violations of the divine order can only be dissolved with the help of God. Everything else is illusion. It is an apparent dissolution <u>without</u> sustainability.

Note 6: If the load is not dissolved by that way, so the cutting of all negative entanglements may be requested. These entanglements can be **centuries or millennia old.** They possibly can be caused by memberships in dark unions, by black-magical methods, by wrong oaths, by curses or other disastrous deeds.

Note 7: Furthermore, we can hand in promises to our future behavior towards God.

Note 8: But woe to the one who is not honest in this just to get rid of his loads quickly.

Note 9: All of us may assume that we are not able to hide anything from God.

Note 10: A hesitation (e.g. at a promise) on our side is enough not to let us

„out" in turn. Then the whole process was a pure waste of time.

Note 11: And if somebody thinks to be able to continue like before after the occured relief, despite of his promises, he then shouldn`t be surprised about all the negative events in his life.

4.6.6.5 Alternative ce): „To be in paradise" by concentration on a picture

Steps	Restoration
ENT	**Entry** like in example **ENT1 + ENT2**
FOC	**Focusing** like in example **FOC1 (F1-F5)**
CLE	**Cleaning** like in **chapter 4.4.3.**
DIA	**Diagnosis steps** like in **chapter 4.5.3.**
RES-II	**Main steps:**
R1	„I concentrate on the picture „To be in paradise".
R2	„ I now let the picture take effect on soul, mind and body and ask for…" (e.g. unity with God).
SEC	**Transmission:** like in **chapter 4.7.1.**
EXI	**Exit:** like in **chapter 4.8.**

Note 1: The **title** of the picture is „**To be in paradise".**

Note 2: To picture contemplation see chapter 4.1.3 e).

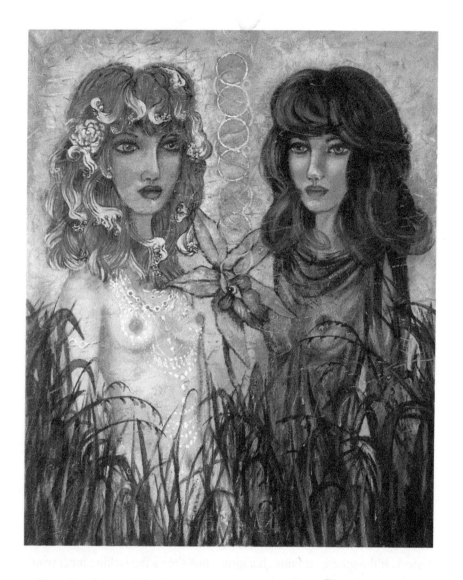

Künstler: Sergey Jelezky, Aus der Serie „Paradies“, Öl auf Leinwand, 100x80cm, 2013

4.7 The Securing Phase

4.7.1 The partial Steps of the Securing Phase (SEC): Version 1

Steps	Securing
SEC1	„Light connection, please, **from forefinger <u>left</u> to the little finger of the right hand.**"
SEC2	„"I pull the scenarion from the **forefinger <u>left</u> to the right side up to the little finger of the right hand** and transmit it to infinity for the eternal further development."
SEC3	„Place, date, time." + Impulse

Note 1: The securing takes place by the little finger right to the infinity.

Note 2: To give the impulse in SEC3 by the little finger right.

Note 3:. It is important that we don`t forget the attributes „place/date/ time" and „infinity".

Note 4: It is also important that the <u>right</u> impulse is given here. If the impulse will <u>not</u> be given, then the sphere stays with the scenario at the right little finger. If only a „<u>halfhearted</u>" impulse is given, then the sphere often flies only very slowly or it even remains „hanging" in some distance from the finger.

Note 5: If the sphere remains „hanging", this shows the lacking inner readiness to take this issue to the right way. That can cause that the session will have to be stopped.

Note 6: This kind of securing contains exactly 3 effects:

a) The sphere near to the body contains all connections to all systems of the world.

b) The transmission to infinity provides the fast realization.

c) The infinite further development provides the consideration of the information in everyone and everything.

4.7.2 The partial Steps of the Securing Phase (SEC): Version 2

Steps	Securing
SEC4	„**Light connection**, please, from the **forefinger right** to the little finger of the right hand.“
SEC5	"I give the **additional order** to the **original sphere** to supervise and guarantee the proper function of all placed spheres. From now on to eternity.“
SEC6	„Now I pull the **original sphere** of the **forefinger right to the right side up to the little finger of the right hand** and transmit it to infinity for the eternal further development.“

Note 1: This kind of securing becomes necessary depending on exercise, e.g. at the creation of an own space/time area.

Note 2: Such an „**interim securing**“ transfers the arranged to safety. That doesn't replace the proper, general exit from the „session“.

4.8 The Exit Phase (EXI)

4.8.1 The partial Steps of the Exit Phase (EXI1)

Steps	Exit
EX1	„I **give light** to this guidance with the light of the Creator, according to the gauge of the Creator, in front of the background of the Creator's soul."
EX2	„I **fix** the result with the light of the Creator. NOW." + Impulse
EX3	„Place, date, time." „I **transmit** to infinity." + Impulse

Note 1: Speak in an incantation manner as this kind of talking is the Kabbalistic form. This is stronger than speaking aloud.

Note 2: To give the impulse in **EX2** by forefinger right.

Note 3: The transmission to infinity is fundamentally important. [31)]

This transmission in **EX3** takes place via light connection to the little finger right and by putting it into infinity (∞) via the little finger right.

Note 4: Although with that each session is completed, but the total task is not yet accomplished. The AFTER-phase is of considerable importance.

Note 5: The „fixing" means the „transmission to all systems in the world", since the light of the Creator is omnipresent.

4.9 The After-Phase (AFT)
4.9.1 The Observation (AFT1)

Note 1: The after-phase applies to the observation.
Note 2: In the after-phase 3 <u>variants</u> show themselves:

<u>**Variant a):**</u> **For easier issues** an improvement arises relatively fast.

<u>**Variant b):**</u> Due to the attached correction in the holistic body the so-called „initial aggravation" arises. **Here the question arises whether the aggravation is really an aggravation or whether it just feels like it to us.**

The <u>development</u> of a real <u>aggravation</u> is e.g.:

Slight problems → heavy problems → death of an area in the body
(with pain)

The <u>development</u> for a correction in the direction of <u>health</u> is:

Death of an area → heavy problems → slight problems
(with pain)

<u>**Thus:**</u> It is clear that a revitalized area could bring „pain" with it at first. So we go 2 times through the pain.

<u>**Variant c):**</u> **Nothing happens.**

Here the question arises whether really nothing happens. The earthly oriented person may notice nothing, but the clairvoyant usually sees the change in the mental, astral or etheral body. Finally it is easy to understand that a problem which was built up e.g. for 20 years mostly cannot lead to the immediate disappearance.

Because: The change of thoughts brings the change in the astral, brings the change in the physical. This can take time.

But if the clairvoyant also sees nothing, then it has to be proceeded according to chapter 4.6.6.4. If this information massiveness is cleared out, then usually something happens as experience shows.

4.9.2 Protection Build-up (AFT2)
4.9.2.1 Alternative a): Protection on knee level

Note 1: The method is shown by Svetlana Smirnova12) graphically very well.

Note 2: If the clairvoyant fixes a problem in the future (that is a problem which advances to a person), then we can still remodel the problem, but no longer protect ourselves against it.

Note 3: Therefore a preventive protection in form of suitable signal transforming reflectors makes much sense. This protection reflects the negative signals, it derives them.

Note 4: Who is not really able to imagine this reflector, should cut e.g. a tomato and practice with it.

4.9.2.2 The extensive Protection

The extensive protection arises by right, fast thinking. 8)

It is explained by commentary to this in chapter G V) in the „Practical Directory for the Technologies and Methods of Grigori Grabovoi". 31)

Thus: „If we lay in a CD of healthy thoughts in our head, then the cells regenerate into living, he althy cells."

Bibliography

1) Svetlana Smirnova:

„Methods of Healing through the Application of Consciousness", general

2) Svetlana Smirnova:

„Methods of Healing through the Application of Consciousness", chapter 8

3) Svetlana Smirnova:

„Methods of Healing through the Application of Consciousness", chapter 9

4) Svetlana Smirnova:

„Methods of Healing through the Application of Consciousness", chapter 13

5) Svetlana Smirnova:

„Methods of Healing through the Application of Consciousness", chapter 20

6) Grigori Grabovoi: „Unified System of Knowledge"

7) Grigori Grabovoi: „Unified System of Knowledge", chapter 2

8) Grigori Grabovoi: „Unified System of Knowledge", chapter 6

9) Grigori Grabovoi: „Practice of the Control", Volume 2 (German edition)

10) Grigori Grabovoi: „Practice of the Control", Volume 3 (German edition)

11) Grigori Grabovoi: „Joy of the eternal Development"

12) Svetlana Smirnova: „Introduction to the Methods of Grigori Grabovoi"

13) Svetlana Smirnova: „Introduction to the Methods of Grigori Grabovoi"

(Technology of the way out of problem states)

14) Grigori Grabovoi: „Restoration of the Matter of Man by Concentration on Numbers", Volumes 1 + 2

15) Grigori Grabovoi: „Restoration of the human Organism by Concentration on Numbers",

16) Grigori Grabovoi: „Concentration Exercises"

17) Grigori Grabovoi: „Educational System of Grigori Grabovoi"

18) Grigori Grabovoi: „Applied Structures of the Area of creative Information"

19) Arkady Petrov: Trilogy „The ‚Creation of the World"

20) Hugin Munin: „Practical Directory for the Technologies and Methods of Grigori Grabovoi", chapter GVIII

21) Hugin Munin: „Practical Directory for the Technologies and Methods of Grigori Grabovoi", understanding key 4

22) Hugin Munin: „Practical Directory for the Technologies and Methods of Grigori Grabovoi", understanding key 5

23) Grigori Grabovoi: „Unified System of Knowledge", chapter 7

24) Grigori Grabovoi: See in his creations to „Raising"

25) Hugin Munin: „Practice Manual with Checklists + Examples for the Controlling of private Projects, professional Projects and also by Companies on the Basis of (Business) Numbers by Grigori Grabovoi."

26) Grigori Grabovoi: „Number Sequences of psychological Standardization"

27) Grigori Grabovoi: „Unified System of Knowledge", chapter 12

28) Hugin Munin: „Practical Directory for the Technologies and Methods of Grigori Grabovoi", chapter G XI

29) Grigori Grabovoi: „Selected Lectures" in chapter „Teaching about the Rescue and harmonious Development"

30) Grigori Grabovoi: „Numbers for a successful Business", chapter: „Types of Business Management"

31) Hugin Munin: „Practical Directory for the Technologies and Methods of Grigori Grabovoi"

32) Grigori Grabovoi: „Selected Lectures"

33) Grigori Grabovoi: „Unified System of Knowledge", chapter 8

34) Svetlana Smirnova: „Workshop for advanced Stage" (Output of the cancer cells through the sky perspective)

35) Svetlana Smirnova: „Workshop for advanced Stage"

36) Grigori Grabovoi: „Numbers for a successful Business"

37) Svetlana Smirnova, "Introduction to the Methods of Grigori Grabovoi"

Lightning Source UK Ltd.
Milton Keynes UK
UKOW06f0750010714

234303UK00006B/6/P